Praise for *Teaching Yoga*

I highly recommend Donna's latest offering, *Teaching Yoga: Exploring the Teacher–Student* Relationship. Donna has consistently worked to bring insight and awareness regarding ethical standards and violations of them within the Yoga community. My prayer is that every Yoga teacher-training program offer a course on ethics, using Donna's book as the text. Upon entering a Yoga studio, students should know that this book is available as a resource and guide for ethical behavior.

—Richard C. Miller, Ph. D, author of
Yoga Nidra: The Meditative Heart of Yoga (book and CD)

Donna Farhi shows that teaching yoga requires both commitment to personal practice and integrity in relationships with students. Her inspiring book is an essential resource for the new generation of teachers who will carry forward this transformative lineage and impart the living experience of yoga to a world in need of healing. Highly recommended reading for anyone who loves yoga and wants to share it with others.

Greg Bogart, Ph. D., author of *The Nine Stages of Spiritual Apprenticeship:
Understanding the Student-Teacher Relationship*

At last, here is a book that dispassionately discusses the ethics inherent in being a yoga teacher in a modern Western context. I recommend this book because it explains the psychodynamics of the teacher–student relationship in ways that show core values, such as respect and fearlessness. But I like this book because it dares to ask us hard questions about living a spiritual life, so that we can teach with clarity and compassion. An instant classic!

—Judith Hanson Lasater, Ph. D., P.T., author of
30 Essential Yoga Poses: For Beginning Students and Their Teachers

Across the millennia, Yogis have recognized that the relationship between teacher and student is central to the transformational potential of yoga. And yet, in the twenty-first century, we have had little dialogue about the precise nature of this relationship. Now—at last!—Donna Farhi brings us a carefully articulated examination of the complexities of teacher-student relationship. *Teaching Yoga* is an exquisitely crafted and important contribution to what should be a lively dialogue in the world of contemplative practice.

—Stephen Cope, author of *The Wisdom of Yoga:
A Seeker's Guide to Extraordinary Living*

Wow! What a thoughtful, detailed, wonderful book. The teacher–student relationship is fundamental to the transmission and teaching of Yoga, and Donna addresses this potentially amazing relationship from many, many angles. This is a very engaging read. Donna presents the fundamental premise, treating others as you yourself would like to be treated, with sensitivity, respect, and the distilled experience of many years on the job.

Erich Schiffmann, author of
Yoga: The Spirit and Practice of Moving into Stillness

TEACHING YOGA

BY DONNA FARHI

The Breathing Book

Yoga Mind, Body and Spirit

Bringing Yoga to Life

Teaching Yoga

DONNA FARHI

TEACHING
YOGA

EXPLORING THE TEACHER–STUDENT RELATIONSHIP

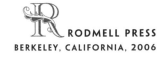
RODMELL PRESS
BERKELEY, CALIFORNIA, 2006

Library of Congress Cataloging-in-Publication Data

Farhi, Donna.
 Teaching yoga : exploring the teacher–student relationship /
Donna Farhi. — 1st ed.
    p. cm.
 Includes bibliographical references and index.
 ISBN-13: 978-1-930485-17-4 (pbk. with cd : alk. paper)
 1. Hatha yoga—Study and teaching. I. Title.
 RA781.7.F373 2006
 613.7'046071—dc22

                                            2006014960

Printed in China

First Edition
ISBN 10: 1-930485-17-4
ISBN 13: 978-1-930485-17-4

10 09 08 07   3 4 5 6 7 8 9 10

Editor: Linda Cogozzo
Associate Editor: Holly Hammond
Indexer: Ty Koontz
Cover and Text Design: Gopa & Ted2, Inc.
Author Photographer: Murray Irwin, Christchurch, New Zealand
Lithographer: Kwong Fat Offset Printing Co., Ltd.

Text set in Renard3
Distributed by Publishers Group West

TO MY STUDENTS,
WHO HAVE BEEN GOOD TEACHERS.

CONTENTS

Acknowledgments   xiii

Introduction   1

PART I   7

UNDERSTANDING THE TEACHER–STUDENT RELATIONSHIP

The Sacred Role of the Teacher   7

What Is a Yoga Teacher?   9

Yoga Teacher as Mentor   15

Ethics and Ethical Behavior   17

Archetypes: How the Teacher Lives in the Student's Mind   20

Yoga Teacher as Healer   22

Yoga Teacher as Priest   25

Yoga Teacher as Parent   26

Yoga Teacher as Lover   30

Transference, Countertransference,
Projection, Adoration, and Emulation   33

Disenchantment with the Teacher
and Renegotiation of the Relationship   35

Healthy Boundaries   37

The Teacher's Social, Personal, and Sexual Needs   47

Summary   49

PART II   51

THE ETHICS OF TEACHING YOGA

Teacher Training   54

Training Programs   54

Certification   60

The Dangers of Charisma and the Pitfalls of Fame   63

Medical Concerns and Making Unfair Claims   66

When to Send a Student to Another Teacher   71

Class Numbers   75

Class Numbers for Workshops and Intensives   76

A Word About Amplification   79

Ethical Class Structures   80

Class Levels   84

How We Communicate with Students   88

Adjustments and Touching   89

The Power of Words   92

Codes of Etiquette   94

Boundaries   105

The Ethics of Money   110

Refunds   119

Work-Study and Scholarships   120

Appropriate Dress for the Teacher   123

Appropriate Dress for the Student   126

Foul Language   127

Confidentiality   128

Speaking about Other Teachers or Methods   131

Ethical Codes   134

Protocols for Handling Complaints   140

Opening Doors   143

PART III   145

TEACHER'S WORKBOOK: RESOLVING ETHICAL ISSUES

A Working Model   145

Stages of Intervention   146

Sample Ethical Inquiries   148

Appendix: Yoga Sutra of Patanjali Sourced   155

Notes   165

Permissions   167

About the Author   169

From the Publisher   171

Index   173

About the CD   178

ACKNOWLEDGMENTS

MY HEARTFELT THANKS go first and foremost to the publishers of this book, Linda Cogozzo and Donald Moyer. Their encouragement to write this book, and their support over two decades of teaching, have been instrumental in shaping my view on the importance of ethics in the Yoga community. I am thankful to all my teachers of Yoga, who each in their own way modeled what it means to be fair and kind. To my dear friend and colleague Dr. Richard Miller, thanks for standing with me. His clarity and willingness to oppose injustice within our community (even at the risk of being unpopular) has given me great solace. I am particularly grateful to the Yoga Research and Education Center for lending their superlative code of ethics to this book. Their personal and professional advice to me regarding the Yogic interpretation of values has been invaluable. Thank you to the women in the Yoga community who shared their stories, for their courage in coming forward with the truth. They gave voice to the immeasurable damage that is done when a teacher betrays a student. Their frustration, anger, and despair helped galvanize my efforts to transform my own disheartenment into positive action. It is incalculable how much my Yoga colleagues worldwide have given me through the demonstration of their own lives and through their honesty. Those who support and host my teaching visits worldwide have given me a platform from which to share the great gift of Yoga. And last, though they may seem unlikely sources of wisdom, to Braga and Tuscany (now passed) and

Numen and Liberty (my current equine companions), for never failing to uncover what is unfinished and unresolved within me. It is good to have two friends who never let me get away with anything!

INTRODUCTION

I BEGAN PRACTICING YOGA at the age of sixteen, when it was offered as an elective subject at my high school in a rough part of South Auckland, New Zealand. In those days, Yoga was considered rather a bizarre practice and especially uncool for a teenager. While throngs of students signed up for ice-skating, swimming, and other alluring elective topics, a handful of misfits, myself included, showed up for their first Yoga class. My "yoga" teacher was actually a physical education teacher with no formal training in Yoga, other than a book, *Richard Hittleman's Yoga: 28-Day Exercise Plan*. She was in the last stages of her pregnancy, so the class lasted only six weeks, but by then I was totally transfixed and had already begun a daily practice at home with the help of Hittleman's book. Such was my commitment to the practice, that when the class ended, I requested that I be able to practice my Yoga alone in a tiny concrete room off the main auditorium during elective time. The principal, convinced I must be doing it as a guise to play truant, hauled me into his office one day, like the cat that had finally caught the mouse. It was only after my homeroom teacher swore that Yoga was exactly what I was doing during elective time that I was able to continue undeterred.

From the very first class I was astounded to discover that such a simple practice as moving the body slowly, counting the breath, or meditating while gazing at a candle could conjure up a feeling of "okayness" within me. Since being moved from America as a ten-year-old girl, my childhood had been characterized by a feeling of fear, uncertainty, and isolation. I received little or no guidance from my parents and had few friends, due to a strong antiforeign sentiment in New Zealand at that time. As I moved into my teenage years, I suffered from a deep sense of depression and desperation, which eventually manifested in anorexia. Because of all these factors, my Yoga practice became a lifeline, and my time alone practicing became an oasis of sanity. Perhaps because I felt so desperately alone and alienated within a culture so unlike that of my origins in America, teachers, then and throughout my life, were to have for me a powerful guiding influence. The teachers who helped me during those first years in New Zealand—the sensitive teacher in high school who prevented me from slipping into oblivion and one special advisor at university—became key guides along the path. During my years studying as a dancer, there would be a special ballet mistress who, even after I had returned to the United States, came to watch me take class and give advice on my progress, though by then she was quite elderly.

At the age of twenty-three, I began my formal study of Yoga and within a short period of time encountered both good teachers and extraordinarily bad ones. After practicing Yoga with essentially no guidance for seven years, without a single injury or a single instance of feeling strain from my practice, within three months of "formal" instruction I had herniated a disc in my neck. After coming down out of a Headstand (Sirsasana) and reporting that I felt pain in my neck, my teacher demanded I go "right back up" and practice an advanced variation, Twisted Headstand (Parsva Sirsasana), which I had no preparation to do. Believing that the teacher must know more than I did (which is what makes a teacher a teacher and a student a student), I obeyed her instruction. The resulting injury left me in severe chronic pain, requiring years of intensive physical therapy and causing a lifelong fragility in my cervical spine. This singular incident would radically shape my own pedagogical model: in my future choice of teachers, how I would teach my own students, and now how I train others to become Yoga teachers.

It was clear to me, even at the age of sixteen, that Yoga is a potent and life-transforming practice. I feel indebted to all the good (and also the very bad) Yoga teachers I have encountered, because one can learn as much from a bad teacher as from a good one. Because I have always held Yoga as sacred, I always considered that teaching Yoga would be a professional practice, to be taken as seriously as training to be a doctor, a therapist, or a priest. It was also clear to me that this would be a lifelong study. Because I have experienced in my own life, and witnessed in the lives of my students, the power that this practice has to both heal and harm, I know that teaching Yoga carries enormous responsibilities. In what other profession must one take into account the physical, psychological, physiological, emotional, and spiritual condition of an individual, and speak to all these dimensions in the course of teaching?

My desire to write this book arises from two sources—the love and respect I feel for the Yoga tradition and the power it has to help people become happy and free, and a sincere wish that students being introduced to Yoga receive these teachings in a safe and sacred environment. There are few places in the modern world where it is possible to do the work of deep transformation. The integrity of the Yoga studio and the integrity of the teacher–student relationship need to be protected as if they were an endangered rainforest or threatened species. There may be more people practicing Yoga now than at any other time in history. While this is potentially a wonderful thing, it also seems that we have never been so close to jettisoning the very spirit of the tradition—the ethical precepts that form the foundation of Yoga, and the foundation of a peaceful life, not just for you and me but for all people. The spirit of the Yoga tradition lies in one central truth: we are all inextricably connected. We are all one community, drawing our breath from the same effulgent source. This awareness of community, or *sangha*, calls us to consider all forms of life with reverence and respect. Respect for life and for others lies at the heart of ethics. Although the subject is complex, I believe ethics can be simply defined as treating others as you wish to be treated yourself.

My work in ethics goes back to my years as a board member of the Iyengar Yoga Institute of San Francisco and of the California Yoga Teachers Association (which at that time governed the nonprofit magazine *Yoga Journal*). I continued this work as a codirector of a school in New Zealand, and more recently as a traveling instructor and leader of Yoga teacher training programs. In my fourteen years of residency in San Francisco, ten of which were spent within these boards, I worked to bring ethical issues to the forefront. One incident was pivotal to my dedication to the issue: a group of colleagues and I tried to prevent a teacher from continuing to harm his students, after receiving reports from women throughout the United States that they had been abused while attending class with this teacher. The reports made me aware of the immeasurable damage that occurs when a student's trust in her teacher is betrayed. The teacher, who had a known and self-admitted predatory pattern of sexually molesting students, and who, in any other profession, would have been barred (and probably imprisoned), continued to be hosted by Yoga centers from coast to coast. As I traveled and taught throughout the world, I often heard accounts of abuse of power, which led me to believe that these were not rare instances but common occurrences. Women who were abused heard of my work, and I began to receive letters, e-mails, and phone calls from them, some of whom were still hurting a decade after their relationship with their teacher had ended.

What astonished me then, and continues to baffle me now, is that these events took place in a time when other professions had made great headway in establishing their own ethical codes and reinforcing these through the legal system. These events took place when our society had already determined that a university professor would be promptly removed, should she be found to have had a romantic alliance with a student; a psychotherapist would be sued for preying on the vulnerability of a client; a doctor would be barred from practicing for misconduct with a patient. In our workplaces and in the educational, medical, and legal systems, we were becoming clear about ethical and unethical professional behavior. But it was not the case within the Yoga community. (The lack of an agreed-upon ethical standard may be directly linked to the absence in most countries of national formal standards to determine professional competency for Yoga teachers.) Teachers with limited training may not perceive of themselves, and the potential effect of their work, in the same way that doctors or psychotherapists perceive of themselves. Another reason for the confusion about ethical standards is because we often assume that behavior within a spiritual context falls outside typical societal norms, and offensive behavior is less so because it carries a spiritual stamp.

By the time I left the United States to return to New Zealand, I felt disheartened by what appeared to be the fruitlessness of trying to promote ethical awareness within the Yoga profession. I decided to turn my feelings of frustration toward a positive goal: sensitizing, educating, and opening up dialogues about ethics within the worldwide Yoga community with this book. In taking on this task, I became acutely aware of my own shortcomings, and in the year of writing this book I encountered some of the most difficult ethical quandaries of my career. I would like to be clear that I do not claim to have an impeccable track record, nor am I immune to ethical mistakes. I still find myself asking, Is this the right thing to do? Could I have handled that matter more skillfully? What will be the outcome of my actions, both for my students and myself? And like all human beings, I often fall well short of the mark. Even so, prior to writing this book, I decided to refuse to teach at Yoga centers that continued to knowingly host teachers with unresolved unethical behavior. And I am beginning to see some changes that give me hope.

The book is organized in three parts. Part 1 addresses the complex nature of the relationship between the teacher and student. Through better understanding some of the more subtle and hidden aspects of this relationship, both teacher and student can make more measured decisions. But my interest in ethical issues within the Yoga profession is not only about the teacher–student relationship but about such matters as the integrity with which we advertise our work, how we teach a group of beginning students, and how we handle monetary issues. The largest portion of the book, part 2, addresses these more practical and equally important aspects of teaching Yoga. As you will discover, there is considerable overlap between the relationship that has formed between the teacher and student and the kinds of ethical considerations that arise in the everyday running of a Yoga studio. Part 3 is a workbook for teachers with exercises for considering common ethical quandaries and the interventions possible at each stage of their development.

Throughout the text, you'll find inquiries to stimulate your own investigation of what it means to be ethical. The inquiries are situations that either have happened to me directly as a teacher or student, or have been passed on from a colleague, peer, or student, or have been contributed by one of my senior students. Contributed inquiries are told in the writer's own words. While the thoughts and conclusions of these inquiries do not necessarily represent my own, they offer valuable insights. All names of teachers and students have been changed to protect privacy. The ethical conclusions are by no means definitive, and your questions and judgments may differ from mine. They are designed to provoke thoughtful debate, for yourself, with your colleagues and peers, and between yourself and your employees.

This book was written primarily as a guide for new and seasoned Yoga teachers, and it is my hope that it will become a resource for Yoga teacher training programs worldwide. I believe the book will also be useful to serious Yoga students wanting to get the very best from their studies. May it be of benefit to all.

—Donna Farhi
Christchurch, New Zealand, 2006

PART I

UNDERSTANDING THE TEACHER–STUDENT RELATIONSHIP

SUTRA 1.1

Now, when a sincere seeker approaches an enlightened teacher, with the right attitude of discipleship (viz., free of preconceived notions and prejudices, and full of intelligent faith and receptivity) and with the right spirit of inquiry, at the right time and the right place, communication of yoga takes place.

THE SACRED ROLE OF THE TEACHER

WHEN I WAS THIRTEEN I had a teacher, Mrs. Buntings, who recognized my sensitivity and creativity and encouraged me to sing, write poetry, draw, and perform. While demonstrating a clear command for her charges, Mrs. Buntings also had a rare ability to balance discipline and order with flexibility. A sunny day might be cause to put our books aside and walk down to the river for a drawing lesson. She encouraged creative freedom when we wrote poems, balanced by the opportunity to learn correct grammar, spelling, and punctuation. The unpredictability of my home life left me feeling emotionally at sea, but within moments of being in Mrs. Buntings' classroom, I felt that I was in a safe harbor. I can't remember a single word that Mrs. Buntings said to me, only the feeling of knowing how much she cared for her students and that I was one of those lucky people who received her benevolence. At the end of two years of intermediate school and on the eve of our departure for high school, her students sat on the step outside her bungalow classroom. Some of us wept at the thought of leaving our teacher, and she, sitting among us, wept too. Mrs. Buntings probably never knew the great solace she gave me just through her very existence.

Years later a very unconventional teacher, Ray Worring, rescued me from the precipice of a breakdown. Having grown up in the big sky country of Montana, Ray could easily have been mistaken for a rancher, but in truth he was a shaman in disguise. Trained as both a geologist and a psychologist, and recognized as a world-class psychic, Ray liked to take his clients "into the field," as he put it, dressed in his requisite cowboy boots and hat. Ray saw that I needed to strengthen what he called my "fragile center." He offered to help me when my life was in ruins, and for an entire week, from dawn till dusk, he took me on a kind of vision quest to help me move beyond self-limiting beliefs and habits into a new, liberated state of being. In the ensuing years we worked together to break new ground and to solidify the lessons learned in those early meetings. Through his consummate skill and infinite care, he brought me back to life. Had it not been for the intervention of this teacher, I would probably not be teaching others today. Ray was deeply moved when he discovered that I dedicated my first book to him. Like all great spiritual mentors, Ray took great pleasure in seeing others become free. Even though he has since passed on, his spirit inspires me to continue helping others as he so generously helped me.

Most people have had at least one special teacher who has influenced her life. And if this influence was a negative one, that simply underscores the most important point of this book: all teachers—math teachers, English teachers, or Yoga teachers—have an ineffable power to bring forth or to destroy the nascent and fragile abilities of an individual. Therefore the role of the teacher is vested with huge responsibilities and equally satisfying rewards. This transformative role can never be fully realized without a safe and sacred environment in which the integrity of both the teacher and the student are sustained.

SUTRA 1.13

The practice of yoga is the commitment to become
established in the state of freedom.

WHAT IS A YOGA TEACHER?

Yoga is a centuries-old spiritual tradition, science, and art that proceeds from the knowledge that all life is interconnected. When we perceive ourselves to be cut off, alone, or separate from life, we suffer. As a consequence of our false perception, our actions in the world may be ignorantly misguided, causing unnecessary pain to ourselves. Yoga tells us that we can disentangle ourselves from this morass of suffering and also prevent suffering for others by recognizing that there is no "one" and no "thing" that is separate from us. We achieve this unitive state not through blind faith or mechanical observance of rituals but through a no-nonsense practice of the eight limbs of Yoga (Ashtanga Yoga). The eight limbs consist of moral codes for living ethically (*yamas* and *niyamas*), somatic practices (*asana*) that bring us into the truth of our embodiment, and breath awareness practices (*pranayama*) designed to resynchronize our individual rhythm with the primordial rhythm of the universe. Through consistent practice over a lifetime, we learn to recognize what is really important and to let go of impermanent objects and transient thoughts and emotions (*pratyahara*). Through this recognition of what really matters, we learn to concentrate our mind and life (*dharana*) on those things that are of lasting value. With practice we learn to maintain our equanimity in the most difficult of circumstances (*dhyana*) and thereby liberate ourselves to reach our highest potential (*samadhi*). As wonderful as all this may sound, Yoga is not a spiritual tradition suited to theorists or those who are inclined to reclining positions. Yoga is for those who have discipline, tenacity, and devotion. It is a pragmatic science where everything is tested and verified through direct experience.

To comprehend the special dynamics that occur between a Yoga teacher and a Yoga student, it is crucial to understand the unique nature of the subject being taught. Yoga is not simply information that the teacher carries and disseminates separate from herself, to be left in the classroom or studio at the end of the workday. What is being taught is a state of being, a way of living, which by necessity is intrinsic to the character of the teacher. In the study of Yoga, the teacher can lead the student only as far as she has gone herself. She can point a light only into places that she herself has been willing to go. She can empathize with the student's spiritual quest, and the issues that may arise during that quest, only because she herself has embarked on such a journey. For this reason, it is difficult to separate the professional life from the personal life of a Yoga teacher. How can a way of life and a state of being be turned on and off at whim or divested when it is convenient to do so? To truly embody the essence of the teachings of Yoga they must, as Patanjali suggests in his Yoga Sutra, be practiced as "universal moral principles, unrestricted by conditions of birth, place, time, or circumstance" (Sutra II.31).[1]

While it is normal in many professions to distinguish between professional behavior and behavior that is permitted in personal life, the profession of teaching Yoga does not permit such convenient bifurcation. The underpinnings of the Yoga tradition have to do with leading a moral life in which our actions are congruent with our values. When we remove the conservative overtones that now surround the word *morality* and consider morality as behavior that reflects a reverence for life, we come closer to the true meaning of morals. After all, everyone wants to be treated with fairness, kindness, and respect. This is only possible when our actions are guided by sound moral principles.

Regardless of the particular style or tradition of Yoga we may be teaching, all Yoga traditions share a common value: that the essential nature of each individual is intrinsically whole, good, and free. The yogic precepts for ethical living, the yamas and niyamas, are emphatic declarations of this inherent goodness, which is apparent whenever the illusion of separateness falls away. The yamas are constraints that we observe in relationship to the world. These are the practice of compassion for all living things (*ahimsa*), commitment to the truth (*satya*), not stealing (*asteya*), sexual propriety (*brahmacharya*), and not coveting or grasping (*aparigraha*). The niyamas are concerned with our relationship to self and how we live when no one else is watching. The niyamas are an important testing ground for whether our private and public lives are congruent and that we walk our talk. The niyamas consist of the practice of purity and cleanliness in body, mind, and speech (*shaucha*), contentment (*santosha*), disciplined use of our energy (*tapas*), self-study (*swadhyaya*), and surrender to God or to the higher Self (*ishvarapranidhana*). Our infinite nature is characterized by the expression of the yamas, or "outer observances," and the niyamas, or "inner observances," when it is emancipated from the confines of the limited identity of the individual.

Patanjali tells us that our true nature consists of these ten qualities of goodness. When we are centered within our true nature, these qualities shine forth. Because of their central importance, the yamas and niyamas are listed as the first two of the eight traditional limbs of Ashtanga Yoga practice, and adherence to these observances precedes and supersedes all other practices. Given Patanjali's logical and systematic presentation of the Yoga Sutra (196 aphorisms that delineate the process of becoming whole), we can be assured that it is not by happenstance that these observances are given such a prominent position. The precepts range progressively from a scrutiny of how we relate to others to an intense investigation of the state of our inner life. Often seen as a list of dos and don'ts, or interpreted as a series of commandments, the yamas and niyamas are actually *descriptions of a nature that has been freed from the illusion of separateness.*

These inner and outer observances are often referred to as the inner and outer "restraints." What we restrain however is not our inherent badness or wrongness but our tendency to see ourselves as separate. It is this tendency that causes us to act outside our true nature. When there is an "other," it becomes possible to do things like steal, because we falsely believe that what happens to another is not our concern. But when there is a sense of unity, who is there to steal from but ourselves? When we feel connected to others, we find that we are naturally compassionate (ahimsa), and that the first yama of not harming is not something we strive to be but something that we are. *Ahimsa* is usually translated as "nonviolence." Unfortunately, in Western culture the word *violence* is associated with extreme versions of behavior, such as physical violence and killing. But this precept calls us to look at nonviolence from the broadest perspective, from the quality of our thoughts and words to our everyday interactions with others. The practice of compassion encompasses the broader meaning of ahimsa as an attitude of nonharming to all sentient beings. We see the essence of ourselves in the other and realize that the tenderness and forgiveness we so wish to have extended toward us is something that all humans long for.

The second yama, truthfulness (satya), is based on the understanding that honest communication and action form the bedrock of any healthy relationship, community, or government. When we feel connected to the vastness of life and are confident of life's abundance, we are naturally generous and able to practice the third yama, not stealing (asteya). This yama expresses itself through generosity and open-heartedness. The fourth yama, sexual propriety (brahmacharya), tells us to use our sexual energy in a way that makes us feel more intimate not only with our partner but also with all of life. When we are connected to our Divinity, how can we use another for our own selfish desires or hurt another through our inability to contain our desires? Finally the fifth yama, not grasping (aparigraha), tells us that letting go of all our embroidered images and identities is a sure way to realize the open nature of the heart. We are told that, even if identities and roles are a necessary part of our everyday life, when we recognize them for what they are, they need not encumber us, and they can never be a true reflection of our absolute nature.

The inner observances, or niyamas, act as a code for living soulfully. They tell us that when we are true to the highest expression of ourselves as humans, we live with purity (shaucha). With a body that is healthy and a mind that is clear, we are more able to practice the second niyama, contentment (santosha). We find that all we need lies within the moment, even if that moment is difficult. This contentment arises out of a realization that no matter how sticky and difficult life can be, when we stand in our center, our inner self remains essentially untouched. To remain centered in this awareness takes discipline and enthusiasm, and thus the fire or heat of spiritual practice (tapas), the third niyama, becomes a way of constantly clearing our slate of the daily residue that can color our perceptions. All these practices require and encourage self-reflective awareness (swadhyaya), the fourth inner observance. The turning of awareness inward reminds us time and again that the authentic life we are seeking is as close as our nose. Finally we can accomplish and live as an expression of all these attitudes when we celebrate the very fact of our aliveness and surrender to life and to God (ishvarapranidhana).

The Yogic precepts are valuable guidelines for living when considered as a whole. Just as the limbs of a baby grow in relation to each other, the eight limbs of practice grow out of the body of the precepts. When we take a single precept and separate it from the support and context of the other precepts, we will be unable to clearly perceive an issue from its broadest perspective. Not-lying (satya) must be balanced by not-harming (ahimsa). There are occasions when telling the truth, especially when it is intended to punish, is an act of violence, and should therefore be censored. The desire to lead a contented life (santosha) is not accomplished through complacency and sloth but rather through the context of discipline (tapas). These counterbalances can activate the process of an internal process of inquiry in determining rightful and wrongful behavior.

As anyone who has attempted Yoga practice knows, it is a many-layered process fraught with challenges, distractions, and roadblocks. We are likely to encounter our worst fears, our most ingrained false beliefs, and our most frustrating self-destructive habits. As Yoga teachers we attempt, through whatever understanding we have gained from our own experience, to act as ushers for the student's fiery process of transmutation. It is our task to ensure a safe and effective context for this process to occur, using skillful means to ignite and sustain the fires of transformation, and providing ongoing support and recognition of the student's intrinsic wholeness, regardless of where they are in the journey. Perhaps this last is most important of all, because when we feel truly seen and recognized we experience profound healing.

In a sense it is through the mirror of the teacher's search for and commitment to his own authenticity that the student gains permission for her innate being to shine forth. Yet the teacher will undoubtedly fail at times; this is part of being human. What is most important is that the teacher has a sincere aspiration and deep commitment to the ethical precepts. All people can and will make mistakes, and both teacher and student need to accept this fact. A teacher who fails, recognizes the mistake, and makes every attempt not to repeat the mistake is demonstrating a groundedness in his own humanity while aspiring to the highest possibility. In admitting a mistake, he is expressing a truth about where he is in his own journey. The balancing of the two polarities of humanity and divinity within the teacher's internal process is an important mirror for the student's process. If the teacher presents a glittering rendition of himself that does not accurately reflect his faults and foibles, or if he denies or attempts to cover up his mistakes, the student may experience alienation from her own shortcomings. Of course the recognition of human limitations is not an excuse to behave badly or a justification (as in "He's only human") when the individual has no intention of changing his behavior. Being human is not a loophole.

If we profess to be teaching Yoga, which is a science and art of living, we must practice that way of living ourselves. If we wish only to teach poses or postures, it would be better to call what we do by a name other than Yoga.

SUTRA 1.40

The sovereignty of the mind that is settled extends from the smallest of the small to the greatest of the great.

YOGA TEACHER AS MENTOR

Because of the special nature of the role of Yoga teacher, the more mature or experienced teacher takes the role a step further and acts as a mentor. In Homer's epic poem *The Odyssey*, the mentor acts as an advisor to Odysseus in his ten-year attempt to return home to Ithaca after the Trojan War. Odysseus's adventure, characterized as it is by hardship, setbacks, and seemingly endless wanderings and near triumphs ending in disappointments, is an apt description of the yogic path.

A mentor is someone who, through her wisdom and experience, sees who we are and has a strong desire to facilitate the blossoming of our fullest capacities. When does a teacher become a mentor? When a teacher has gained the absolute trust of the student, and this feeling is mutual, the relationship between teacher and student becomes very close. Both parties become invested in the most positive outcome, with the student seeking advice and gaining insight that can often only be drawn from such a senior source. The transition between viewing the teacher as an instructor and as a mentor may take place unconsciously, but once this transition has been made there is usually an unspoken recognition and appreciation for the preciousness of the relationship. How precious a gift it is when anyone, whether friend or mentor, recognizes another's unrealized potential and is sincerely invested in the manifestation of that potential in a healthy and life-giving way.

A mentor draws forth what is in the student's imagination and helps him to define what may appear vague and illusive. A mentor assists the birthing of the student's dreams, visions, and hopes, and most important, what the student has not yet dared to imagine. A mentor moves the student from disbelief to belief and in the process continually affirms the student's self-worth. In the best possible scenario, a mentor passes on the torch of her knowledge while at the same time encouraging the student to become his own person. Ultimately the mentor is the embodiment and mirror of the student's own wisdom nature, pointing the student toward his inner teacher, known in the Yoga tradition as the *atman*. The atman is a latent and effulgent source of wisdom that is only fully liberated when we begin to trust in our own direct insight. A true mentor does not cultivate the student's dependence on her insight but facilitates the student's trust in his own inner promptings. This is the beginning of independence and true freedom.

One of the characteristics to look for in a mentor is someone who takes great pleasure in the smallest improvement in her student. This satisfaction is completely altruistic and is an expression of the Yoga teacher's self-sufficiency and self-realization. A mentor expresses the third *brahmavihara* (quality of heart) (see Sutra 1.33), which is to see and celebrate the good in others and celebrate another's success as your own. This quality of heart becomes firm in those whose own ego is stable and balanced. The teacher's own identity structure is secure and is not dependent on putting the student in an inferior position. When a teacher does not have this healthy ego structure, she may express envy, jealousy, or covert anger when a student's progress surpasses her own development. Commonly such a teacher will attempt to knock the student down a notch or two by undermining his confidence. Obviously this benefits neither student nor teacher. A student who later became a Yoga teacher described to me how her own teacher exhibited dismay when she expressed a desire to attend a Yoga teacher training. The teacher exclaimed, "You? Why would you consider attending a Yoga teacher training?" Such was her humiliation in the face of such opposition that she shelved her plans to attend a training for many years. This student is one of the most intelligent, enthusiastic, and disciplined I have encountered and a clear candidate to become a Yoga teacher, so I can only surmise that her former teacher felt threatened by this student's accomplishments. Likewise, if a Yoga teacher cultivates a particular student because of what the teacher might gain, either personally or professionally, through increased status or financial reward, the relationship will always be tainted by the teacher's desire to complete herself through the student.

SUTRA II.29

> Discipline, observances, posture, exercise of the life-force, introversion of attention, concentration, meditation and illumination (at-one-ment) are the eight limbs of yoga or the direct realization of oneness. Hence, these limbs should all be practiced together, intelligently, so that the impurities of all the physical, vital and psychological limbs may be eliminated.

ETHICS AND ETHICAL BEHAVIOR

While the moral precepts presented by Patanjali in his Yoga Sutra offer us a system of values, each is presented as a skeletal structure open to individual interpretation. We flesh out the sutras through practice and our direct experience born from taking (or not taking) certain actions. The brevity of Patanjali's descriptions of the moral precepts has, unfortunately, given rise to a great deal of liberty being taken in their interpretation. There is no clear consensus within the Yoga community as to what constitutes ethical and unethical behavior. So what can other professions offer us in their interpretation of ethics?

In *The Ethics of Caring: Honoring the Web of Life in Our Professional Healing Relationships*, Kylea Taylor defines the terms: "Ethical behavior is reverence for life demonstrated by right relationship to another."[2] Jesus said it even more simply in urging his followers to "Do unto others as you would have them do unto you."[3] "Rachel Naomi Remen in her article *On Defining Spirit* says that 'ethics is a set of values, a code for translating the moral into daily life.'"[4]

Taylor suggests that, besides considering ethical standards, one also needs to be operating from what she calls an "internal locus." When our internal locus for ethics is fully engaged, we will continually understand what is ethical in a particular situation, with a particular person, at that particular time and place. For instance, it might be ethical to physically hold someone who is grieving and has asked to be held. The same behavior might be unethical if a student has expressed romantic interest in us, and close physical contact is likely to confuse the student further. Similarly it might be ethical to invite a student to lunch to discuss his difficulties in a training course, and it might be unethical to accept an invitation to go to dinner with a student if the invitation appears to be a sexual overture.

While an internal locus is crucial, the external locus provided by a code of ethics, whether this be the yamas and niyamas or a code set down by a professional organization, is also important. The external locus gives us a structure from which to consider our actions and a starting point from which to ask important questions. The external locus provides a center, a group, an organization, or a community with a clear consensus about shared values. The external locus, especially when it is part of a prerequisite agreement (as when a Yoga teacher signs a contract to work at a center), helps to prevent serious deviation from ethical behavior caused by personal interpretation or manipulation of an agreement to suit the individual, especially when those deviations are selfishly motivated. The external locus also gives those in a leadership role a clear contract with employees, which may be used as a starting point for discussion or used to break the agreement when conditions are not met. A code of ethics, such as those of educational, medical, and psychotherapeutic professions, also allows a professional body to act as a clearinghouse for ethical concerns and complaints, so they can be handled in a responsible way. When no clear agreement exists (as is true in many contemporary Yoga centers), directors leave themselves open to their employees radically deviating from the values they hold for their center and their students.

Still more important, the external locus provides a context for considering what is ethical and a platform for the deeper inquiry required when considering the internal locus. For instance, because I know it is unethical to steal, that may inform my decision-making when setting fees and may ensure that I cover the material I agreed to cover in a class. The external locus (not-stealing) gives me a starting point for engaging a deeper process of discernment, so that I might waive fees for a student with serious medical problems, while insisting upon prompt payment from financially able students. If I inquire more deeply, I might decide that waiving a fee for someone in great need prevents me from stealing, while asking students to pay fees promptly prevents them from engaging in a form of stealing. Further inquiry may show that fees provided by financially able students help to support those less fortunate. The external locus of a code of ethics provides a window into the deepest and broadest perspective on what it means to live an ethical life.

When we are not certain whether a behavior or course of action is ethical, we might ask ourselves these questions:

- Would I like to be treated in this manner myself? How would I feel if this happened to me?
- How will I feel about this later? Am I comfortable telling others or having others know about my actions?
- Has this behavior in the past required me to betray, lie, or practice any other form of subterfuge or cover-up? Would I be likely to act untruthfully in the future if I repeat this behavior?
- Is this action likely to create suffering for me or another person, either in the short term or the long term?
- If I were a student in this Yoga class, how might I perceive the actions of my teacher? For instance, if you were a student in an intensive and noticed that the teacher gave one particular student more attention than

anyone else or shared every meal with a student, might you feel that the teacher is displaying favoritism? Might you suspect that the teacher is hoping to develop a personal relationship with that student? As someone who paid the same fee to attend the course, would you feel that you had been treated fairly?

- Is there a discrepancy between my stated value and the way that I feel about that value? For instance, your stated value may be that you do not give refunds for class cards that are not used by the expiration date, but when you have to enforce this you feel guilty. What shift, either in your stated value or within yourself, would allow you to feel an agreement between your external action and your internal process?

Sutra 1.4

In the absence of the state of mind called Yoga, the ability to understand the object is simply replaced by the mind's conception of that object or by a total lack of comprehension.

Archetypes: How the Teacher Lives in the Student's Mind

As teachers, we need to look not only at how we consider our role as teacher but also how we live in the student's mind. It can be surprising to learn how large a part we sometimes play in the student's experience. Often the seemingly casual student who we barely notice in class may see us as a lifeline. We may even have a huge impact on students we have never met, who have studied our work through books or videos. For this reason, we should never underestimate the impact of our words and actions. Throughout my many years of teaching, letters from students have awakened me to the immense impact a teacher can have. Here is a sampling of those letters.

"I am aware of a heavy burden of loneliness, of carrying a weight, and of how seldom I meet anyone with whom I can share anything as freely, perhaps because you are not afraid to be yourself, and that is what I notice most of all."

"You taught me more about living and myself than any other person in my life . . . without that I don't know if I would have been able to make it through the emotional pain I was in last year."

"Since reading your book I have become qualified as a Yoga instructor and feel that my life is finally heading in the right direction."

"I confess that at the healthy age of sixty-six this is my first letter to a mentor, and a young one at that."

"The reason I decided to study with you this year is the first time I saw you at a conference I thought you were really stuck up. I took an immediate dislike to you. Such was the strength of that reaction that I wanted to investigate why you push my buttons."

"Obviously fame and fortune have gone to your head and this is why you were so distanced from me during the last Yoga intensive."

Few professions encompass as many roles as that of a Yoga teacher, and thus we may live as a complex arrangement of archetypes in the student's mind. (An archetype is a universal yet usually unconscious idea, pattern of thought, image, or belief that is present in the individual psyche.) It is unlikely, for instance, that someone would assume that an engineer would be an ideal source for medical advice, or that a genetic scientist might also pass as a marriage counselor. At any given time, however, a Yoga teacher may act in a capacity similar to a teacher, doctor, psychotherapist, physical therapist, priest, cheerleader, parent, or beloved. What all these roles share is an implicit imbalance of power based on the trust invested in the teacher. Whenever someone seeks the assistance of another person, whether for education, therapy, counseling, spiritual guidance, or medical, legal, or financial advice, there is an asymmetrical balance of power because one person carries the valued knowledge and skill. This inequity is set up by both parties: when we establish ourselves in such a role and when the other person perceives us in that role.

I recently spoke with a colleague about his sexualizing behavior in relationships with students and teacher trainees. He attempted to both justify his behavior and relinquish responsibility for it by saying, "I am not a spiritual teacher. I am a friend to my students." Yet in his advertising he describes himself as "a Yoga master." Few of us would describe our friends as our masters. The word *master* means "a person with the ability or power to use, control, or dispose of something,"[5] and in this context it means an adept or expert. Clearly there is confusion here between his self-designated title, and what a student might assume from the title, and his wish to renounce his responsibilities. This would be deeply confusing for a student. As one of his female students put it, "He told me that when I am in the classroom I am a student, and outside the classroom I am his lover. It's that simple!" But our emotional structure is not that simple. Few people can turn their feelings on and off at will, and if they can it is often to the detriment of their own emotional integrity.

There are specific reasons why some roles are particularly potent in the case of Yoga teachers. Let us look further at a few of the possible ways we live in the student's mind.

Sutra II.15

Life is uncertain, change causes fear, and latent impressions bring pain—
all is indeed suffering to one who has developed discriminations.

Yoga Teacher as Healer

The archetype of the healer contains many subsets: doctor, physical therapist, psychotherapist, shaman, and more. These roles assume specific skills that have the potential to heal and to engender hope of healing in the client. Many practitioners call themselves Yoga therapists and actively solicit students who have acute or chronic physical problems. Yoga teachers often do work similar to that of a doctor. We work with debilitating back problems, serious illnesses such as cancer and cardiovascular disease, and many other conditions, many of which have not been ameliorated through other modalities. What is more, some of us spend far more time working with our students (within each session and over the long haul) than doctors are able to. Of course, I do not mean to imply that standard medical care should not be obtained or is insufficient. But most medical consultations are brief and infrequent. It is not uncommon for patients to see a different doctor on each visit, with little continuity of care. On the other hand, Yoga students usually have regular contact with their teachers, sometimes spending years, if not a lifetime, together.

In the early years of my career, I developed a special-needs Yoga course for students who would otherwise have been unable to practice Yoga, even in the most elementary class. Many of my special-needs clients were referred from local physical therapists, postsurgery spinal units, and other practitioners, such as chiropractors. I occasionally gave in-service teaching sessions to physical therapists working at the hospital. And I began to ask myself this question: If I am working in a capacity similar to a physical therapist or doctor, should I not hold myself to similar professional and ethical standards?

My university academic advisor (who was himself interested in alternative healing) used to say that a person's belief in a healing method was almost as important as the treatment itself. He also believed that people go to therapists, doctors, and other healers as much for the quality of presence they receive as for the expertise. When I began my own private practice as a bodyworker and Yoga teacher, I found both these premises to be true. Clients would often comment that the pristine order and calm of the treatment room made them feel immediately better. I also noticed that my own choice of health practitioners depended on the ability of those healers to focus completely on the process and to listen carefully to my concerns. In considering the archetype of the healer, we should be mindful that giving our complete presence and attention to a person is healing in and of itself. What we offer is encouragement and faith in a person's capacity to heal, never promoting the notion that we, as teachers, are the dispensers of healing. As a student gains mastery in offering herself unconditional attention and commitment to healing practices, we should make it clear that it is the student's connection with her own inner wisdom that ultimately heals.

ETHICAL INQUIRY:
PUTTING THE TEACHER ON A PEDESTAL

While teaching a workshop in Britain, I asked a student's permission to adjust her Yoga posture and whether she would mind if the group observed our work together. She agreed to work with me, and as we began I noticed that she was visibly shaking. "Are you alright?" I asked. She immediately came out of the posture and admitted that she was very nervous and was "shaking with fear." I asked her if she felt self-conscious demonstrating in front of the group. "Well no, that's not it. It's just that it's Donna Farhi adjusting me!" I replied, "'Well, you know, I feel like a very ordinary person. I put my pants on one leg at a time, and although it might be hard to fathom, I even go to the bathroom!" The group laughed, and the tension lifted. When I later reflected on this interaction, I realized how this woman had built me up in her mind. I imagined that to her being adjusted by me was the equivalent of meeting the prime minister. How she perceived me made it difficult for her to learn in my class. Although I can't control how someone else perceives me, this and similar incidents have caused me to reflect on ways that I might self-disclose as a means of humanizing myself to new students.

Self-disclosure should never take the form of the teacher revealing personal affairs, but when self-disclosure is used to elucidate a teaching point, it can both clarify the point and increase the empathy between student and teacher. For instance, as a passionate horsewoman, I often tell my students how frightened I was to work with one of my spirited young horses. I described how, instead of walking away from that fear, I broke down the process into a series of incremental steps, slowly building the skills I needed to overcome my fear. In telling my students that I still feel fear, I humanize myself and also demonstrate that while fear isn't something to be denied, neither should we turn away from it.

As a student, notice how putting a teacher on a pedestal affects your ability to see the teacher clearly and inhibits your ability to learn. As a teacher, notice if you enjoy being put on a pedestal. How does it feel to be considered important? Is your sense of self-worth dependent on the adoration of your students? ■ ■

SUTRA II.26

Ignorance is destroyed by the undisturbed discrimination between the Self and the world.

YOGA TEACHER AS PRIEST

A priest is someone who stands with us in our greatest moments of doubt and acts as a keeper of the faith. Our students may hold us in their minds and hearts as such guides. They may confess secrets, fears, and wounds that they have told few others. A student may tell us of his diagnosis of cancer before telling his wife and children. Another student might share the shame he feels in having a mental illness, having kept this secret from his friends and workmates all his life. And still another student might tell of her lifelong struggle with alcoholism, bulimia, or sexual addiction. Students invest enormous trust in us, and we must keep that trust by holding confidentiality. In the same way that a priest in a confessional booth is sworn to secrecy, confidences shared should be held in trust unless otherwise agreed. Students often share confidential information with us because they are too frightened or ashamed to share it with anyone else. They may feel that no one else would understand or hold such information with care. It may even be necessary to assure a student that we will hold anything that they tell us in trust.

The student may also see the Yoga teacher as the one that holds the container of the sacred space in which he can explore his connection to his Divinity, to his atman (inner teacher), or to God. For many people, having a place in which they can explore their relationship with a higher power, and speak openly about their spiritual path, is a rare gift. For some students the Yogic relationship may be the only context in which they feel free to discuss their spiritual journey. Working with the archetype of the priest involves not only bearing witness to the student's process but encouraging the student to find her own steadfast inner witness. Learning to access this interior priest or priestess helps the student to find her own power to invoke sacred space and draw upon resources of higher wisdom in times of need.

SUTRA II.24

It is ignorance of our real nature that causes the Self to be obscured.

YOGA TEACHER AS PARENT

Whether the student imagines the teacher as a literal mother or father figure or, more broadly, as an expression of the universal mother or father, this archetype is a common projection between student and teacher. We are authority figures who are also caretakers, so students often project their undigested childhood experiences and the relationship they had with their parents onto Yoga teachers. This process can be amplified when the student finds herself in a residential retreat or intensive that in some way mirrors a home environment. For that reason, I discovered early on that it was a good idea when working intensively with a group to have both a male and a female teacher present. As one colleague put it, "That way there is a Mommy and a Daddy, and both instructors can share the fallout of projections!"

One of the common expressions of this archetype is the desire of the student to be taken care of by the Yoga teacher and an unconscious desire for the teacher to amend for the perceived lack of care or attention received in his childhood. Additionally there may be a strong need for approval, recognition, or reassurance of self-worth, especially if these were lacking during his upbringing. Sometimes the archetype manifests in displays of rebellion, much as we might see with a teenager pushing the boundaries. As Yoga teachers, we can make it clear that while we will make every effort to care for the student, we will not take care of the student, lest we infantilize him and promote an unhealthy dependence on our attention. While we may offer praise and acknowledgement, when these are sought in an attention-getting or needy way, it is important to facilitate the internalization of self-approval, self-soothing, and self-worth processes. It has been my experience that when a student acts rebelliously, reactively, or inappropriately, he generally has had a chronic problem with boundaries as a result of insufficient boundary-setting during his upbringing. In these cases, the Yoga teacher needs to be absolutely confident in presenting clear boundaries, upholding those boundaries, and if necessary offering a consequence to repeated crossing of boundaries.

I once had a student who always arrived at least fifteen minutes late and sometimes as much as forty-five minutes late for class. This woman would travel halfway across the country for a workshop and then be late for class, even though her room was just down the corridor. After requesting that she attend on time (or not at all), and having this request repeatedly ignored, I asked the receptionist at the Yoga studio to refuse her entry should she arrive late again. Not surprisingly, she badgered the receptionist, making all kinds of excuses and qualifications to enter, and predictably the receptionist caved in. One could almost see her as a child, whining and badgering her mother until her mother gave her the candy, let her go to the dance, or bought her the dress she wanted. I was not willing to disrupt the class to address her entry, because she came in during a crucial practice. Finally, one day she arrived forty-five minutes late, and I whispered to my teaching assistant to ask her to leave the class immediately without engaging in any discussion with her, other than to say that the only condition of her entry to class was that she come on time. You might imagine how unpopular an action this was, but she never showed up late to class again.

Whenever a student has a strong or inappropriate reaction to a situation, I am suspicious that something from the person's past is triggering the reaction. The trigger may be deeply embedded in her subconscious as a residue from childhood. I recall a particular female student who requested a meeting with me after a class to vent her rage (alternating between anger and bouts of sobbing) about how I only criticized her practice and never praised her. At the time I was taken aback by her reaction because all I could recall was spending quite a bit of time helping her with a particular pose. Then I realized that my correction of her pose must have provoked a strong memory of criticism from her childhood in which, as she put it, she could "do nothing right." When I asked if she would be willing to explore her reaction with me, it became clear that this was indeed the case.

The teacher needs to be mature enough to recognize when a process of projection is in full swing and not take the student's reaction as a personal attack. Staying calm, nondefensive, and detached, while making it clear that we do care, provides a centered place from which the student can slowly extricate herself from the projection and see through to the source of the reaction.

One of the most powerful ways that we can work with this archetype is to turn the student toward the ultimate source of care, the Universal Self. As the student learns how to connect with and trust in her larger Self, she can truly move into adulthood. This can have life-changing consequences in the student's intimate relationships: no longer seeking a father for a partner, no longer seeking a mother for a partner, she is now free to enter into more liberated adult relationships.

ETHICAL INQUIRY:
PUSHING THE BOUNDARIES

Kevin attended a residential Yoga teacher-training course and within minutes of arriving at the venue was raising the eyebrows of my coteacher and the assistant teachers in the dining hall for his inappropriate comments to me. He presumed an arrogant familiarity that lacked respect and proper teacher–student decorum. Over the course of the next few days, in teachers meetings we labeled him a "special-attention person" and designated an assistant who had bonded with him to keep tabs on his behavior in class and to offer support as needed.

It quickly became apparent that Kevin was not only in the habit of crossing boundaries with his teachers but with the other trainees. One participant told how he walked up to her table after dinner, picked up her teacup, and took a sip! Another complained that he had added his clothing to her load of laundry without asking her. One day I discovered that he had taken my compact discs back to his room and burned copies without my permission. Within days internal arguments and factions formed as a result of his behavior. His aggressive and defensive communication style was expressed in many ways: in scathing commentary about others, in inappropriately revealing clothing, in showing up late to class, in cutting people off midsentence or contradicting their perceptions during teaching practicums.

The teachers met to decide what should be done, and my coteacher and I arranged to meet with Kevin to present our concerns and to see whether he would be willing to recognize and work to change these behaviors. We were prepared to suggest that Kevin spend twenty-four hours considering the suitability of the training for him and whether he was willing to work with his behavior, and if not to leave the training and receive a refund for the unattended sessions. As has happened on a number of such occasions, Kevin preempted our move, announcing the following morning that he had decided to leave the training. Not surprisingly the other attendees expressed relief at Kevin's departure.

After many Yoga teacher trainings, I now can recognize the signs of a student whose dysfunctional patterns are so ingrained that they cannot work effectively within a group. Such students most likely will require many years of one-on-one therapy with a trained professional. We should not be reluctant to ask such students to leave when their behavior is so disruptive that it negatively impacts the group and when their behavior cannot be addressed successfully in a group setting. ▪ ▪

SUTRA II.38

Through communion with God, one becomes truly strong.

YOGA TEACHER AS LOVER

It may seem peculiar to include the lover archetype here, but there is nothing more intoxicating to many students than the attention of their teacher (and vice versa). You may be the first person who has truly seen the student, and the student may then begin to see himself as special. You may be the first person to show unqualified concern and care, to listen attentively when she speaks. Indeed the Yoga teacher is attempting to practice an unconditional presence at all times. Should it surprise us then when a student reads into this relationship the possibility of intimate union? It is possible for both the teacher and student to hold fantasies about each other. There is nothing inherently unwholesome about sexual attraction and the fantasies borne on the heels of that attraction. When these feelings are contained and not acted out, they can be harnessed for the benefit of both parties.

It is difficult to know whether this phenomenon is stronger in women than in men, given that most Yoga classes are predominantly female. There does appear to be a high incidence of women, especially young women, seeking a sense of self-worth through intimate relations with their Yoga teacher. I have listened to the stories of many such women, all of whom seem to share a poorly developed sense of self that caused them not only to seek out an intimate relationship with their male Yoga teacher (most often married) but to continue the relationship long after it had proven a source of conflict and suffering. As one woman described it: "Each encounter gives me an initial high, followed later by a sense of deep worthlessness."

The subject of appropriate boundaries and ethical teacher-student relationship is discussed in depth later in this book. For now we can see this archetype as the ultimate universal longing—a yearning for deep intimacy and belonging. It includes the desire to cherish and to be cherished, to see and be seen. When a teacher understands this archetype for what it is—a desire on the part of the student to reconnect with her higher Self and to feel whole within that self—then he can understand the gravity of holding the boundaries between himself and the student secure.

We've looked briefly at the archetypes of the healer, the priest, the lover, and the parent. This brief list is certainly not exhaustive and other influences certainly do exist. How a teacher lives in a student's mind is impossible to predict or to quantify. Therefore it is always safer and wiser to assume that we live in the student's mind in a larger way than we can imagine. Following on this assumption then, there is an even greater responsibility to hold the integrity of the relationship.

Before we discuss the ethics of the teacher-student relationship further, it may be helpful to look at some of the common phenomena that inform interactions between the teacher and student.

ETHICAL INQUIRY:
SEXUAL CONQUEST

It was not hard to notice that Chris, while serious about his Yoga study, also seemed to take every opportunity to use class as a possible meeting place for potential girlfriends. The end of a long weekend workshop could see him with several young ladies, heading out to the nearest café. Young female students flocked to him like bees to honey. While Chris seemed to irritate my teaching assistants, I had had a discussion with him over dinner one night that helped me to develop greater compassion for him. He shared how he had left home at a very young age and had to grow up fast, so he missed out on the fun and carefree years of childhood. He perceived becoming a man and having a stable, committed relationship as a threat to his freedom. And, if I were brutally honest, I also noticed a certain girlish flutter in myself when he was around. He could be very charming and had a strong sexual charisma that could not be denied. I simply observed these feelings within myself, neither suppressing nor expressing them. Observation of my feelings allowed me to recognize my own need for feminine acknowledgement. More important, observation of these feelings allowed me to recognize the potential for using a student for my own needs and therefore helped me to be particularly conscious of my boundaries with him.

But then one day, a number of weeks before a teaching engagement, Chris contacted me, wanting to take me out to lunch prior to the workshop, or better yet, to be my tour guide for the day. While all of these offers might have been entirely innocent of lascivious intentions, I couldn't help wondering whether even unconsciously Chris was looking for another conquest. I declined his invitations but suggested that we make time to talk about his practice over the weekend. I made a point of speaking to him at the end of class, commenting on the changes in his practice, praising him for how much he had integrated since our last time together, and listening to his questions. Most of all I wanted to let him know that he was seen: not seen as a young male, not seen as a possible lover, but seen for his essential self. I wasn't interested in trying to change Chris's promiscuous behavior but rather to offer him an alternative way of interacting with women. The jury is still out on what consequence these interactions will have for Chris. As the teacher, however, my ability to maintain a clear personal boundary in one arena, while opening up a transpersonal connection with Chris, left me feeling very centered. Although engaging in a sexual relationship with Chris or with any student had never been entertained as even a remote possibility, it was an interesting exercise to observe my feelings. I found it even more interesting to imagine how disempowering to me it would have been to take advantage of a vulnerable young man: How pathetic would it be to use someone so clearly unequal in position and power? And, of course, how ultimately disempowering it would have been for him.

In listening to my story, you may want to reflect on how you, as a Yoga teacher, handle the feelings that arise in response to sexual attraction toward a student. Reflect without editing your feelings or emotions. As you do this, can you identify a deeper root cause for those feelings? How might you meet yourself and have your own needs met outside the context of the teacher–student relationship?

SUTRA 1.4

At other times, when yoga does not happen and when the mind is busily occupied with the movement, there is a cloud of confusion in the undivided, homogeneous intelligence. In the shadow of that cloud, there arises false identification or cognition of the movement of the mind-fragment and hence distorted understanding.

TRANSFERENCE, COUNTERTRANSFERENCE, PROJECTION, ADORATION, AND EMULATION

In Yoga practice we attempt to dismantle the layering of false identities to reveal our true Self. Many of these false identities are formed in our childhood through our interactions with immediate family, friends, and the culture in which we live. The term *transference*, most commonly used in psychotherapeutic settings, refers to the way in which a client may develop powerful feelings toward her therapist, some of which may be a recapitulation of the emotional dynamics within her family past. For instance a Yoga student may flirt with her teacher in the hopes of becoming the "chosen one." This behavior may be an unconscious enactment, based on her past desire to receive her father's (or mother's) approval and attention. She may have learned to seek her sense of self-worth through the approval of men, or through her ability to seduce them. Trying to seduce her teacher may be as much about repeating this past habit as it is seeking a response that will discourage it. In fact if the teacher can maintain a clear boundary at this time, he is offering the student a golden opportunity to free herself from a pattern of behavior that may have caused her significant suffering in the past and may be the source of more suffering in the future. By maintaining clear boundaries while continuing to affirm the student's inherent worth, the teacher may also be offering her an opportunity to recognize her intrinsic wholeness, rather than further fostering the belief that she must complete herself through another.

Countertransference refers to the way a student, client, or patient may evoke repressed feelings on the part of the teacher, therapist, or doctor. For instance the teacher may have a deep and often unexamined need to be important, respected, or to feel that she is a charismatic or popular person. In the ethical inquiry about my student Chris, I was able to identify a process of counter-transference occurring, and this knowledge helped me to be even more care-ful in maintaining a clear boundary. When countertransference does occur, it is crucial for a teacher to have the ability to contain (which is different than suppress) her feelings and to tend to those feelings outside the context of the teacher–student relationship.

Undoubtedly as common and no less confusing is the process of *projection*, whereby each person in the equation projects an assumed idea, belief, or judg-ment and attributes it to the other person. In my book *Bringing Yoga to Life*, I devote an entire chapter to this dynamic because of the way in which our prac-tice of assumption trips us up at every turn.[6] For instance, the teacher may make a cursory judgment that a student is slothful and lazy based on his obe-sity. When examined more deeply, she may come to recognize that these are qualities she self-attributes when she herself feels overweight. She has thus projected her own self-loathing and judgment upon another. On the other hand, a student might project the quality of invincibility upon the teacher, a conviction that nothing can possibly faze him, and be shocked to see his teacher angry, irritable, or ill. The student may have developed a view that Yoga will lead to an idealized state of being, beyond normal feelings, normal reactions, and normal human capacities, and that the practice will provide spiritual insurance against anything bad happening. When we can recognize our projections for what they are and claim them as our own feelings, thoughts, and judgments, we have an opportunity to examine our motives and beliefs and thus interact from a clearer place with others and ourselves.

Adoration and *emulation* are qualities that are not necessarily negative. We may be inspired by our teachers and wish to emulate their good qualities and strengths and honor the gifts we have received from them. Those we admire may have motivated positive actions and directions in our life. This desire however can leave us vulnerable when we ascribe impossible perfection onto our teachers and give them more power than is healthy. How can we differentiate between a healthy expression of honoring a teacher and putting a teacher on a pedestal? When we honor a teacher, we may do so while being fully aware of the teacher's foibles and faults. When we put a teacher on a pedestal, this may obscure our vision of the teacher as a human being. In the process of upholding this perfect picture, we may choose to ignore abusive, manipulative, and even violent behavior in our instructors rather than shatter the idealized world we have created.

DISENCHANTMENT WITH THE TEACHER AND RENEGOTIATION OF THE RELATIONSHIP

After studying with a teacher for a long time, the strong feelings of adulation that characterized the early stages of the relationship can and will change.

When the honeymoon is over, and we discover that our teacher has weaknesses, irritating habits, and frailties—like every other human we know—we may feel disappointment, and even bitterness or betrayal. It's important for both student and teacher to recognize that disenchantment as a normal part of the student's process of individuation. Unless the disenchantment has been caused by unethical behavior or abuse on the part of the teacher, we can view it as a normal and expected process. This is similar to the process we go through as children, when we first realize that our parents are not the superhuman rocks of Gibraltar we took them to be but human beings with feelings, just like us. A mature student will recognize this new point in the relationship and integrate the disenchantment as a transient stage. Similarly a mature teacher will not take such disenchantment personally (for instance, by being crushed when a student decides to study with another teacher) but will see it as a normal process of individuation and exploration on the part of the student. Frequently when a student has moved on to another teacher, the student has learned all she can from us. It can be an awkward time, but it is usually appreciated if the student thanks the teacher for all that has been received and announces her decision to move on to another teacher. When a student has spent many years of study with a particular teacher, this is a respectful way to end the relationship, certainly better than the teacher finding out secondhand that he has been replaced. However, it can be much easier for both parties, and prevent many hard feelings, if the teacher can recognize and anticipate this new level of individuation on the part of the student, praising the student's progress while referring her on to a more senior teacher.

Sometimes disenchantment can cause a student to explore many other teachers, only to return with a new appreciation for her original teacher.

The more considerate one is, the more one stimulates
friendly feelings among all in one's presence.

HEALTHY BOUNDARIES

For the process of transmutation to occur, healthy boundaries need to be
established and sustained by both student and teacher. In the best possible
sense, the teacher acts as a crucible for the student's process of transformation. By necessity a crucible must be of a harder metal than the element that is
being melted. The teacher acts to uphold a safe and sacred container in which
the process can occur. In the same way that discipline limits in order to liberate, containment helps us to narrow our focus so we can gather and concentrate our energy toward a singular purpose and thus be more likely to succeed
in our endeavor. This is apparent even in the physical dimension of containment that is provided by the confines of the four studio walls, and it will be
apparent to any teacher who has tried unsuccessfully to conduct a Yoga class
outdoors and found her students distracted. There are many simple things
that a teacher can do to provide a container for the student's process—beginning and ending class on time, limiting questions to those that are relevant to
the present inquiry, and holding steadfast to the purpose of the practice.

While I believe that maintaining clear boundaries is always the teacher's
responsibility, I also believe that a great deal of abuse in our community
would be prevented if students were to increase their own awareness about
healthy boundaries. Some of this education happens through a teacher mod-
eling clear boundaries. For instance, many students do not even consider that
they have the right to request that a teacher not physically adjust them, or to
ask a teacher to modify they way in which they are being adjusted. When a
teacher asks permission to touch a student in class, she is subtly broadcasting
to that student and to all the other students that they have a right to choose,

and that they have a responsibility to engage a boundary-making process that feels comfortable for them.

While educating students about their choices is not the central purpose of this book, increased student awareness and education is an important component in reducing the incidence of boundary transgression in our community. The changes in our laws and public education about sexual harassment in the workplace has made a generation of women aware that they should no longer tolerate being inappropriately touched in the workplace or any place for that matter. It was the education of the women about their rights that made the most difference in challenging a common behavior and making it absolutely unacceptable. In the same way, I believe student education would go a long way toward reducing the incidence of abuse. Why is it, for instance, that the woman who is touched inappropriately on a bus calls it sexual assault, yet the same woman in the context of a Yoga class is uncertain as to the appropriateness of her Yoga teacher placing his hands on her genitals? Clearly there is the need to educate students that this and other abuses of power and position should not be tolerated. Let me be clear—it is not the student's responsibility to prevent abuse from happening. It is always the teacher's responsibility to maintain integrity in the relationship. The education of students about their rights, however, serves to reduce the chances that once abuse has taken place it will go unchallenged and thus continue.

The ability of a student to form and maintain healthy boundaries is intimately related to the pedagogic model from which the teacher is working. When the teacher is working from a pedagogical model in which the self-sovereignty of the student is the central aim, with all the faculties of self-sufficiency and self-determination that lead to this maturation, students are able to stand in their own center of gravity. When, however, the pedagogical model fosters dependence and a lack of interior reference, the student remains infantilized, unable to engage her own interior reference point, and thus entirely dependent on the teacher to set the boundaries. I've discovered in my teacher training programs that few teachers have examined the underlying premises that determine their instruction or, more important, how these hidden premises affect their relationships with their students. For instance, one of the key premises that underlies my own teaching is a belief that instruction should always be moving the student in the direction of an interior reference point. I am not interested in a student's ability to be obedient to instruction but rather in his ability to inquire into the meaning and relevance of an instruction for him. If I believe a student has the ability to answer a question she has posed to me, I might respond by saying, "That is an excellent question, and I believe you are in the process of answering it yourself. Please let me know what you discover." More often than not, the student comes to a conclusion that is the same as the answer I may have given, but it is now her discovery. This kind of pedagogic model helps students understand that, while I may be an authority in my field, and while they may respect my opinion, ultimately the source of wisdom lies within them. This model serves to foster an intimate process of shared inquiry while at the same time establishing a clear separation in which each participant, teacher and student, remains whole.

For the process of transformation to be effective, a necessary distance is required between teacher and student. We might imagine teacher and student sitting on a seesaw. In order to keep the movement of transformation going, the teacher and student must sit far enough apart to balance each other's energies and to see each other as individually whole. If they come too close together, the movement of the seesaw stops. This necessary distance also magically potentiates the exchange. For instance, when we go to see a priest or rabbi, the ritual acts of dressing for the occasion, traveling to the church or synagogues, and meeting in its sacred confines are ritual elements that elevate the exchange to a higher octave. In the same way, when we go to see a therapist, we may see our time within the office as a special haven where we can uncover our deepest fears and memories. If the context of this exchange becomes too casual, it can undermine what may be possible. For instance, a student may have just had a deep awakening through the practice of Yoga Nidra,[7] Corpse Pose (Savasana), or meditation. It is likely that the student now needs to integrate this experience into the context of his life, work, and relationships. It would be confusing for the student to then become involved with the teacher as a personal friend or social acquaintance. Imagine how confusing it would be if, during a therapy session, you remembered an experience of incest from your past, and afterward your therapist asked you out for a beer and to see a movie! While this may seem farfetched, Yoga teachers often do just the equivalent of this by not understanding the deep process that may be occurring in the student and honoring it through maintaining a necessary formality. The student may feel caught between two worlds: the potent exchange of teacher and student and the often alluring opportunity to have a casual exchange with the teacher. Most often this kind of casual relationship serves the teacher's needs far more than it does the student's.

In the same way, if the teacher considers his role too casually, he can devalue the potential currency of what is possible in the classroom. Whether arriving late, sipping coffee while teaching, or answering the phone during a private lesson, such behaviors can communicate that the exchange is not of great importance or, worse, that the other person's Yoga practice is of little value.

Years ago I learned the hard way about the importance of these boundaries. A group of Yoga students had joined me for a weekend retreat at a center north of San Francisco. One of the features of this center was a beautiful swimming pool, and the manager let it be known that inside the pool gates nudity was permitted and, indeed, encouraged. My then-husband was with me that weekend. Almost all the Yoga students decided to sun bathe and swim naked. It seemed that keeping my bathing suit on was just as awkward a statement as taking it off. I rationalized, naively, that with my husband present, my being naked could not be misinterpreted as a signal of sexual availability. When I returned home from the retreat, however, I discovered an obscene phone call on my answering machine. I recognized the voice as one of my students, whom I'll call Jimmy.

For many months I had been aware that Jimmy harbored fantasies about me, expressed in subtle and not so subtle ways. I was careful in class not to physically adjust Jimmy's poses, and I deliberately used a very matter-of-fact yet cordial tone of voice when addressing him. On a number of occasions, he had asked for a private lesson or stayed after class to ask me to join him for a cup of coffee. Given my sense of his romantic leanings, I had told him that I was unable to take him on as a private student, and I referred him to another teacher for private lessons. I believe I was handling the situation with Jimmy ethically. My hope was that his fantasies would gradually abate and defuse, and that his attentions might be turned more fruitfully to his practice. But this awareness of his past behavior was not at the forefront of my mind that day. Clearly my disrobing at the retreat had sent him into a spin, one that he may have deeply regretted. As it turned out, he was leaving town the next day for a job in another city, and his phone call was a way of discharging the built-up fantasy. However embarrassing and regretful, the experience was also a turning point for me. I recognized that I could not be a teacher and one of the gang at the same time. Given the same situation today, I might request that everyone remained clothed, or I might wait until the retreat was over to enjoy the pool with my husband in private. These decisions would not arise out of prudishness but out of a desire to maintain consistent parameters between my students and me.

Students Who Become Friends

It is inevitable that some of our students will become personal friends. Often this occurs when a student is approaching a peer level with the teacher. Such a shift in relationship should not occur, however, without some serious prior consideration. We might ask ourselves if the opening to the student as friend is primarily a means of getting our social needs met. More important, we might ask whether this change in the relationship will diminish our usefulness to the student and our effectiveness as a teacher. If we wish to be of service to the other person, will this change in the relationship undermine that service? After over twenty years of teaching, I have come to recognize that when a student becomes a personal friend, my ability to serve her as a teacher has effectively ended. When this occurs, it can be helpful to verbalize the change in relationship and suggest that the person find another teacher. When a student has moved into a peer relationship, this may not be necessary. The equivalency of the power dynamic in a peer relationship may make it easier for a person to be a student–peer in class and a friend outside of class. The teacher may also recognize and acknowledge the peer relationship in the classroom, referring to his or her peer in a way that reflects equality within the relationship.

Enmeshment

When an appropriate boundary has been transgressed, it usually causes a clear energetic discomfort. We might think of boundary transgression as someone dismantling the fence around our home. We are immediately alerted that our personal boundaries have been trespassed, and we are clear about the cause. The process of enmeshment, however, is much subtler than this and therefore also potentially confusing. Enmeshment can be difficult to discern because there is almost always a component of manipulation involved.

In "Good Fences Make for Good Relations," author and meditation teacher Phillip Moffitt describes *enmeshment* as "an inappropriate merging of identities" which can be treacherous and confusing to navigate.[8] In enmeshment it's not clear where I begin and end, where the other person begins and ends, and subsequently one or both parties may be unclear about the responsibilities and concerns of that personal identity.

Moffitt writes: "It can take many forms: Your spouse tells you what to think; your sister-in-law shares inappropriate details of her sex-life; your mother corrects the way you speak to your children—in front of the kids;

your best friend tells you whom you should date; your coworker asks for 'help' with her work, but she's really asking you to do it for her; your boss calls you at home to ask you to do the task he has neglected. In each instance, if you can't maintain your boundary, you acquiesce and are pulled into someone else's drama."[9]

In enmeshment we may find ourselves taking responsibility for things that we neither agreed to do nor on reflection want to do. Or we agree to do something but we feel mentally or emotionally in conflict with our agreement. There are three reasons why we may find it difficult to extricate ourselves from a relationship mired in enmeshment. First, while we may recognize that we're uncomfortable, we may not be able to put our finger on the source of that discomfort. Second, we may be unable to accept that we are uncomfortable, resentful, or even angry in response to the enmeshment. Finally, in the case of those of us on a spiritual path, we may wrongly assume that we should feel different, that if we were more generous, more gracious, or more "spiritual," then we would be okay with the circumstance. We may wrestle with our inability to accept our own feelings, and this may deter us from taking any action. When we are able to accept our feelings in an unqualified way, we can take appropriate action to reassert healthy boundaries.

When attempting to determine what is a healthy boundary for yourself, feel into your body and ask these questions:

- When I consider doing (fill in the blank), does this cause energetic discomfort or uncomfortable feelings to arise in my body?
- When I consider not doing or allowing (fill in the blank), what feelings arise in my body?
- Am I unable to assert my boundaries because my primary concern is about protecting, not hurting, or not offending the other person?
- When I honor how I feel in an unqualified way and imagine the outcome that would allow me to respect my boundaries, how do I feel in my body?

ETHICAL INQUIRY:
PRIVATE SPACE

Clarissa maintained a demanding teaching schedule and because of this she had decided not to teach Yoga lessons in her home. This was her way of preserving a sanctuary from the pressures and concerns of teaching. Despite this resolve, due to a complicated situation that had arisen at her studio, she agreed to allow a Yoga student to stay in her home for a week, telling the student that she had reservations about the arrangement. But despite her clearly expressed reservations, she allowed the student to negotiate a stay of three weeks. Although Clarissa was not comfortable with this arrangement, she felt that she couldn't say no to someone in need. Although she did attempt to clarify what she could and could not do for the visiting student, she soon found herself driving the student to appointments and doing other favors that she had neither agreed nor wanted to do. She rationalized that she "should feel okay" about helping another person, but in reality she felt increasingly resentful and angry that she was taking responsibility for someone else's life.

What could Clarissa have done differently to maintain healthy boundaries for herself (and for the student)? ■ ■

SUTRA II.34

Negative feelings, such as violence, are damaging to life, whether we act upon them ourselves or cause or condone them in others. They are born of greed, anger or delusion, and may be slight, moderate or intense. Their fruit is endless ignorance and suffering. To remember this is to cultivate the opposite.

Sexual Ethics

In his landmark book *Sex in the Forbidden Zone*, psychiatrist and teacher Peter Rutter writes: "Any sexual behavior by a man in power within what I define as the forbidden zone is inherently exploitative of a women's trust. Because he is the keeper of that trust, it is the man's responsibility, no matter what the level of provocation or apparent consent by the woman, to assure that sexual behavior does not take place."[10] Rutter further explains that "the forbidden zone" always exists in the relationship between doctor and patient, therapist and client, clergyman and congregant, lawyer and client, and teacher and student, where one person holds in trust the intimate, wounded, vulnerable, or undeveloped parts of the other person.

Although most documented transgressions by Yoga teachers are overwhelmingly perpetrated by men, this is not to say that such transgressions do not occur with female teachers or that women do not hold equal responsibility in their relationships with their students.

One of the most helpful aspects of Peter Rutter's thesis is his definition of the word *abuse,* which is derived from *use* and means "a departure from (Latin: ab) the purpose (use)."[11] When you feel yourself at risk of sexualizing a relationship with a student, you might ask yourself, Am I departing from the greater purpose of my role as teacher? Am I departing from the greater quest, which is to help the student to discover his true identity? If we look deeply at the traditional purpose of Yoga practice, we will see that it is about self-realization, and, most specifically, the liberation of the person from a limited or false definition of self. When the teacher abandons this quest, he essentially removes the context for the student to continue her own spiritual quest.

Teachers should be clear that sexual ethics extend far beyond simply refraining from having sexual relations with students. Sexualizing the teacher-student relationship can take many forms: the way we look at a student or group of students, gestures that we use, our tone of voice, our choice of language, the physical proximity with which we work with a student, the clothing that we wear, and the quality of touch imparted during an adjustment. At a party or social gathering, it is easy to see who is "on the make." Likewise students can easily detect a lascivious intent in a teacher who is using his students to meet his own needs.

Gray Areas

What about the many Yoga teachers and students who have met their partners or spouses through practice? This is a tricky issue, and these relationships should be approached with care. Some useful guidelines that have resulted in lasting and wholesome partnerships are these:

- The teacher maintains a period of withholding from the relationship to examine her projections.
- The teacher discusses the potential relationship with a peer, mentor, or therapist.
- The teacher explicitly ends the teacher–student relationship if both parties agree that they wish to proceed with a more personal relationship. The now exstudent should be referred to another teacher for instruction.

When does a personal relationship begin? As soon as both parties agree that they wish to see each other outside the confines of class, and outside the confines of the teacher–student relationship. A teacher might then say, "If we go out on a date, I can no longer be your Yoga teacher" or "If we explore a romantic relationship, I can no longer be your Yoga teacher."

When both parties are interested in a long-term relationship based on commitment, it is a fundamentally different situation than when a teacher has a predatory habit in class and uses her student base as a resource for casual affairs. These (more serious) relationships often arise when a teacher and a student are close to being peers. It is natural that someone who has chosen Yoga as a life path would want to find someone to share this path. For teachers who live in small rural towns or isolated areas, the choice of partners available to them may be limited. This circumstance should not be used as an excuse, however, and the choice to begin a personal relationship should be approached carefully and with great reservation.

However, and this is a *big* however, it may not become clear until much later how the asymmetrical balance of power that existed between teacher and student prior to their personal relationship may have insinuated itself into the personal relationship and manifested in an unequal balance of power. This unequal balance of power can subtly undermine the integrity of such a relationship.

SUTRA II.37

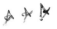 When we are firmly established in integrity,
all riches present themselves freely.

THE TEACHER'S SOCIAL, PERSONAL, AND SEXUAL NEEDS

One of the ways that we, as teachers, can more effectively meet the needs of our students is to make sure that our own needs are being met. This involves making sure that we have the social, personal, and sexual aspects of our lives nurtured and fulfilled. For many teachers, this may involve actively cultivating a social network that is deliberately outside (but not necessarily exclusive of) one's student base. Having friends, peers, support networks, and intimate relationships that are separate from our role as teachers allows us to develop many aspects of our personality that cannot be developed in the teacher–student relationship. Moreover, many aspects of our lives cannot and should not be shared with students, and it is important that we have an outlet to express these aspects of our being. For instance we would feel justly disconcerted if our therapist spent time during a counseling session describing in detail his sexual likes and dislikes. In the same way our Yoga students do not need or want to be privy to detailed information about our personal lives. I believe that the most effective way that teachers can minimize the risk of using students for their own needs, and potentially abusing the students' trust, is to invest diligently in securing a network of support. More important, a teacher who is fulfilled within her own life is more able to give completely and generously to students.

There are many ways to secure a network of support. Teachers, especially those working as independent contractors and beginning Yoga teachers, can benefit by having regular meetings with other teachers. Gathering a small cadre of Yoga colleagues whom one trusts and respects—to practice, discuss difficult students, brainstorm about strategies for successful intervention, or simply to socialize—can be an invaluable source of both personal and professional support. You might also seek the help of a supervisor in a more senior teacher, someone you can consult about issues surrounding your teaching. For instance, one of the key friendships I have cultivated over the years is with a woman who is the director of an acupuncture school. We are in similar positions of leadership, and even though our professional fields are different we have very similar challenges with our students. Being able to openly discuss our frustration, our confusion, or simply our fatigue from the demands of teaching is vitally important in making a place for our humanity, in full knowledge that our discussions are held in absolute confidentiality. Just as you would not want your therapist to tell you how tired or bored she is listening to your problems, it is not appropriate for Yoga teachers to discuss such personal feelings with their students. But there does need to be a place where such feelings and concerns can be aired.

Investing time in maintaining sound personal and familial relationships, as well as broadening one's perspective by forming friendships with those outside the Yoga community, helps insure that when we need support there will be someone to answer the phone, someone to call when we need a shoulder to lean on. Having consciously cultivated such a social network over many years, I have observed that being with friends who aren't solidified around seeing me as a Yoga teacher allows me to let my hair down in a way that is not possible when I am upholding the mantle of the teacher. Having this outside network has also enabled me to become less and less identified or fused with the identity of teacher and thus has created a sense of freedom within myself. I have also discovered that this outside network has given me an interesting perspective on ethical and unethical behavior.

ETHICAL INQUIRY: HAVING A SUPERVISOR

This inquiry was contributed by a colleague.

"I live in a very small town in an area where I've lived all my life. My parents have always lived here too, which means that I know an awful lot of people around here! Many people who I previously knew as friends are now my students as well. Many people who are my students have been very generous in inviting me to parties, dinners, and lunches. My view at the moment is that, yes, I do have to be on my guard, and I believe that a good supervisor can help enormously. For me this is a place where I can go with all the burdensome stuff that is inappropriate to discuss with friends, whether they are students or not. If I start to feel like I'm spilling out all over with worries around my students, I know my session with my supervisor is overdue."

Consider the ways in which you might use a supervisor, mentor, or support group of colleagues. What signs indicate that you are leaking boundaries with your students? ■ ■

Summary

How do we know when the relationship between the teacher and student is healthy and wholesome? Consider this question from both viewpoints: as a teacher and as a student. Teachers can also reflect on how they would answer these questions when they find themselves in a student role. The best teachers continue their education as a lifelong process; being in the student role can offer unique insights into what works and what does not.

As a student, what conditions need to be in place for you to feel safe in your practice? What conditions optimize your ability to learn, to absorb what you learn, and to apply new skills in the context of changing situations? What kind of relationship with your teacher fosters your growth and development as an individual? As you become clear about the answers to these questions, this will inform your choice of teacher and the relationship you wish to have with that teacher.

As a teacher, what conditions allow you to work most effectively with your students? What factors need to be in place for you to focus your energy on the task of teaching without becoming drained and exhausted? What conditions need to be present for you to serve your students while at the same time serving yourself? As you become clear about the answers to these questions, you will develop a model for teaching that supports your values.

As you investigate these questions, doors will open leading to other doors and other questions. From the yogic viewpoint, all these questions lead to an ultimate question: Is my Yoga practice leading me to freedom? When we stand within that freedom, whether as teacher or student, we feel whole within ourselves. We realize that while teacher and student are interconnected, the essence of wholeness is inside each of us, paradoxically independent of each other. This self-sovereignty allows both teacher and student to stand within their own center of gravity.

PART II

THE ETHICS
OF TEACHING YOGA

SUTRA 1.33

The mind becomes clear and serene when the qualities of the heart are cultivated: friendliness towards the joyful, compassion towards their suffering, happiness towards the pure, and impartiality towards the impure.

IN PART 1 WE EXPLORED the permutations and complexities of the relationship between the Yoga teacher and student. But our consideration of ethics must not be confined to that relationship alone. As any Yoga teacher who has had even a modicum of practical experience knows, ethics and ethical decision-making are part of our everyday functioning as Yoga teachers, from how we dress to how we are paid and how we handle complaints about other teachers. In this section we look at some of the practical issues that arise in the course of practicing as a professional teacher. Although many of these concerns may seem mundane, how we handle the everyday matters of teaching is the most palpable and sometimes most potent way that we demonstrate our understanding of and commitment to the ethical precepts of Yoga.

It has been said that only the ethical are encumbered by ethics. If you frequently find yourself pondering the correct or most skillful action in a given circumstance, you are already concerning yourself with the subject of ethics. When you pause to reflect on the consequence of speaking about another person without her being present, you are practicing ethics. When you question your motives in any given situation, you are being ethical. When you consider how someone might feel as a result of your actions, you are being ethical. When you concern yourself with the impact that your personal actions may have upon your community, you are considering ethics in its most pertinent form.

Most people sincerely want to do the right thing. As a Yoga teacher, I travel throughout the world each year to many countries and cultures and work within many Yoga traditions and methods. I notice that teachers who act unethically often do so not because they are bad people but because they simply are not aware of the issues at stake. Most often they do not perceive the larger ramifications of their personal actions, and frequently they have not yet begun the process of discerning that an action, which might be ethical in one's personal life, may be unethical in a professional context. I believe that the foundation for acting ethically lies in thoroughly sensitizing and educating ourselves about ethical issues, so that we might have the broadest possible perspective on what it means to act with integrity, both for ourselves and for our students.

We can educate ourselves in four ways. First, we can start with our own tradition, that is, with the ten ethical precepts for rightful living contained within Patanjali's Yoga Sutra. Second, we can understand ethics in terms of what has already been discovered by other professions, both like and unlike our own.[1] Next, we can look within the larger culture at the laws we have agreed to follow. At times we have to fall back on these laws when our own communities either do not have procedures for resolving conflicts or are inappropriate venues for doing so. Finally and most important, we must be unafraid to assess our deeply held values and how we wish to sustain, uphold, and if necessary defend them. Then, because it is in our best interest and the best interests of others, we are more likely to act ethically.

To be ethical is to realize our complete interdependence with all beings and all living things. It is to know—in the deepest sense that it is possible to know—that everything we think, say, or do has an effect, both on ourselves and on others. If we had already achieved this level of self-realization or uni-tive state (which in essence is the very meaning of the word *Yoga*), the issue of ethics would be moot. But because few of us have attained this kind of absolute clarity, and because Yoga is a lifelong apprenticeship in which our own life is the laboratory of inquiry, the desire to be ethical requires an ongo-ing practice of reflection.

In the interest of simplifying this discussion, I have deliberately separated the subject of the ethics of the teacher–student relationship from the practi-cal, everyday issues of ethical teaching, although inevitably there is a great deal of crossover between these two subjects. Part 1 discusses the dynamics of the teacher–student relationship, not because it is more important but because relationships are complex. How we set up the relationship between teacher and student inevitably has an effect on how we deal with the everyday issues that arise in teaching Yoga. While part 1 looks at the personal conse-quences for both teacher and student, part 2 addresses the communal and public consequences that our actions have upon Yoga as a profession, a spiri-tual tradition, and an art. How do our actions affect the public perception of Yoga, positively or negatively? How can we ensure that what we do today con-tributes to an authentic legacy for future Yoga practitioners?

Having struggled and oftentimes floundered with these issues for over two decades of teaching Yoga, and having arrived at some effective strategies and solutions, I hope that this section of the book will expedite the process for others and give both new and seasoned Yoga teachers a map for traversing the difficult terrain of working as professionals. Teaching Yoga is a minefield of challenges. Let's look at how preemptive and thoughtful action can lead to harmony within our classes and Yoga centers.

Sutra I.14

It is only when the correct practice is followed for a long time, without interruptions and with a quality of positive attitude and eagerness, that it can succeed. (The goal of practice is to bring about a change in the quality of the mind. When practice is pursued for a long time without interruption, and when the results, good or bad, do not bring about elation or dejection, then the practice is considered to be deeply rooted and bound to succeed.)

TEACHER TRAINING

The issue of standards and certification processes, as well as the value of having a regional or nationally recognized registry for Yoga teachers (as is the case in some European countries), is perhaps one of the most controversial subjects within the Yoga community today. Of particular frustration to many highly qualified and experienced instructors is the competition they now face from the plethora of Yoga teachers whose certification can mean as little as a weekend training program. How can we differentiate ourselves as authentic Yoga teachers to a public that has little or no means of discerning the difference? If you are considering training to become a Yoga teacher or obtaining continuing education, or if you are a student looking for an authentic and well-trained teacher, these recommendations may be helpful.

Sutra I.13

The practice of yoga is the commitment to become established in the state of freedom.

TRAINING PROGRAMS

In considering a Yoga teacher training certification program, the first thing to look for is whether the program reflects the broad spectrum of Yoga as a complete spiritual tradition. Many programs teach only the physical dimensions of the practice (asana), with an emphasis on the teacher's ability to do virtuoso gymnastic postures. While this may be impressive among Yoga practitioners, there are few students to whom this will be of great relevance or value. More important, a training program should cover all the eight limbs of practice: ethical precepts for rightful living (yamas and niyamas), the practice of postures (asana), mastery of breath awareness and using the energy of the breath (pranayama), restoration of the ability of the sense organs to perceive the neutral ground of experience (pratyahara), focusing of the mind (dharana), maintaining concentration in meditation (dhyana), and reunifying oneself with the larger Self (samadhi). A training program should also provide some education about the history of Yoga, its philosophical foundations, as well as the various types of Yoga—selfless service (*karma* Yoga), devotional practice *(bhakti* Yoga), (and) conceptual and intellectual study through secular learning and sacred scripture *(jnana* Yoga), to name a few—so that the teacher trainee might consider a form of practice that is suited to his disposition and ability. Such a program might also expose students of a particular tradition to the value of other methods and traditions, such as practices of devotion, service, chanting, or contemplation, as a means to developing respect for those traditions. This can be helpful later, in directing students to methods that may be beneficial.

The second thing to look for in a training program is the length of time required to complete the training. Some things simply cannot be learned in a weekend, in a week, or even in a month. Some skills can only be attained through years of apprenticeship and practice with an experienced teacher. Additionally some aspects of self-awareness, especially as they pertain to our own level of personal integration, can only be uncovered and integrated over time. Generally the better training programs take at least two to three years of study. Most are structured to accommodate participants who need to work, at least part-time. Some are structured with regular intensives throughout the year, and others accommodate those who work full-time by scheduling workshops during weekends and evenings. How a training program is structured may be a crucial factor in your decision-making process. However, even after long training programs, it can take decades to become truly adept at teaching. Those entering training programs should be aware that the end of formal education constitutes the beginning of their work as a Yoga teacher. Serious beginning teachers will continue to diligently pursue their studies—with other teachers, in their own personal practice, and through ongoing self-analysis of the efficacy of their teaching methods.

The third dimension to consider is the quality of the faculty. What kind of training and experience do the teachers have? Are these teachers respected and reputable within the community, as opposed to being celebrities or merely popular? Have they undertaken long periods of study, whether in a traditional ongoing relationship with a teacher or through recognized and respected training programs? In this regard I often recall the advice of one of my mentors: "Go to the horse's mouth; find the best teachers in the world and if necessary travel to study with them." This turned out to be sage advice, because I learned that when you work with a teacher who has very high standards, you tend to reach for a higher goal yourself. When students cannot find an experienced teacher in their area who shares their values, I recommend that they invest in one to two weeks of intensive study with an accomplished teacher each year, rather than continuing ongoing study with a poor teacher with whom they feel a conflict of values. Those intensive periods of study can provide enough material for an entire year of exploration in personal practice.

Next ask what prerequisites are required to attend the training. Increasingly Yoga teacher-training courses are being offered to those who have never so much as attended one Yoga class. It would seem logical that someone wanting to teach Yoga already has some experience in practicing, just as it would follow that you would learn the Spanish language before becoming a Spanish teacher! One to two years of consistent practice under the tutelage of an experienced teacher is a reasonable guideline for such a prerequisite. It would be wise to question the motives of a person wanting to train as a Yoga teacher who has no prior experience, as well as the motives of an organization offering a course with no prerequisites for its participants. I suspect that such prerequisites would both radically reduce the number of people entering Yoga teacher-training programs and the organizations offering such programs.

Another factor in choosing a training program is considering the "reflected value" of the particular Yoga community (*sangha*). My colleague Richard Miller used this phrase often when we cotaught a Yoga retreat last year, and I have since adopted it because I feel that the idea of gathering support and cohesion through shared spiritual practice is one that is sorely needed in our community. Do the members of the center or ashram display qualities of compassion, cooperation, and support for one another? Or is there an atmosphere of fear, competition, and self-defeating one-upmanship? How do you feel when you are with these people? Do they reflect your values? Generally the tone of a center is reflected in the values of its leadership. Time and again I have seen how the clarity and supportive attitude of a strong director attracts similar qualities in the teachers who work at that center and also attracts students who wish to be in such an atmosphere. Similarly I have seen centers headed by egotistical and aggressive leaders who attract similar individuals as their followers. As a Russian proverb says, "A fish rots from the head down."

Finally there is much to be said for doing research. While some research can be done on the Internet, there is no replacement for getting a feel for a place and for the faculty by visiting a center. You may find that attending a national Yoga conference is an expeditious way of trying out a number of teachers and methods. As you narrow down your search, you might then attend workshops with the teachers with whom you are considering further training. Take the time to visit potential training centers and, if you can, talk to other trainees and graduates to get a feel for the level of satisfaction of the participants. As part of your research, compare curriculum perspectives and fee structures as well as the program schedule before making a final decision. This initial research can reduce the chances of locking yourself into a program that might later prove to be unsuitable.

ETHICAL INQUIRY:
BUYER BEWARE

This inquiry was contributed by a colleague.

It began on the Internet, where the Web site proclaimed the existence of The Khandallah Institute, offering a month-long, 200-hour Yoga teacher-training program. Located in the tropics, on the sandy beaches of the Pacific, it claimed to offer clean accommodations, delicious food, and great swimming. My teacher had been invited by the director of the institute to teach three hours each day, and I was to accompany her. It all sounded too good to pass up.

When we arrive we discover that The Khandallah Institute is located on a dead piece of desert, where tents and teepees, trailers and stick shacks spread between the road on one side and the vast Pacific on the other. The ocean here is too dangerous for swimming.

Our accommodation is a tiny trailer with two dirty white plastic chairs outside. It stinks of mildew and is dirty. The trailer is a quarter of a mile away from the two flush toilets and two showers. Our only light is from the candles we brought with us. It is by far the worst place either of us has ever stayed.

When I ask if the 200-hour program is really long enough to prepare people to teach Yoga, the director says, "Probably not. It's really healing we're giving them. They're lost souls and I'm making their lives a little better."

The director's son essentially runs the program, teaching Yoga, meditation, and chanting, dispensing therapy, offering guidance, setting up "vision quests," and supervising the details of everyday life. When I ask him what his background is, he says, "I did some workshops with John Milton. He's an amazing guy. He leads groups all over the world, for CEOs and everything."

"Is he a Yoga teacher?" I ask.

"No," he says, "He doesn't like Yoga."

The Institute schedule begins at 7:00 A.M., with an hour of sun salutations and the director's own form of "flow asana," do the same sequence of six poses each time. The instruction is vague and rambling, filled with dime-store, New Age wisdom. The director had already told us that he never does asana, and his son says the only time he does the asanas is when he's teaching.

The "delicious vegetarian diet prepared by Swiss chefs" that we were promised turns out to be plastic bowls of overcooked vegetables mixed with soy sauce and salad, set out twice a day.

After three days, we realize that things are not going to change. The director lied about everything: the place, the conditions, the food, his own practice, the weather, the outhouses, the lack of electricity, the lack of cleanliness, the lack of preparedness of the students. It was not just the indigestible food, the lack of care, and the ugliness of this place that was so upsetting. What was really intolerable was the total lack of awareness and consciousness in the leaders, reflected in the grounds, in the kitchen, and in what is being transmitted to the students.

On our last day, my teacher meets with the director. He shows up late, still in his bathing suit, his hair wet from surfing.

"So, how has this been for you?" he asks.

She tells him that things have not been at all as he'd led her to believe. As the conversation winds down and no mention has yet been made of money, she says, "I'd like to be paid before I leave."

The director complains, "Money is really tight just now; there's only four thousand dollars in our bank account. We may have to get a job."

"I do retreats all the time, so I know that you should have taken in forty thousand dollars for this month. It can't cost more than twenty to run the program. How could you only have four thousand left? I'd like to be paid before I leave tomorrow."

"I can send you a personal check in a few months."

"I'd like to be paid in cash before I go."

"I tried to get money in town yesterday, but the machine was broken."

"But can't you get money when we go to the airport?"

"I guess that will work," he says, not sounding convinced.

In the end, he did pay her at the airport. Two months after the program ended, the director offered one of the students, his surfing companion, a certification for five hundred hours if she would be his administrative assistant for one of the upcoming sessions. ■ ■

SUTRA 1.21

The more intense the faith and the effort, the closer the goal.

CERTIFICATION

The issue of Yoga teacher certification is one rife with controversy. I do not pretend to offer a definitive answer to this question but would like to open the matter to further inquiry. While it is prudent to err on the side of thorough, supervised training rather than superficial, unsupervised training, even the most rigorous certification programs can produce poor teachers. While technical skills and knowledge can be taught and learned, qualities such as sensitivity, basic people skills, and a natural affinity for and love of teaching are character traits that are not so easily learned. I have met many teachers who have been certified at very high levels but who fail to operate successfully as Yoga teachers because they are simply not good with people. One particular teacher comes to mind; he has moved from city to city, alienating both students and other teachers everywhere he goes and bitterly concluding that it's just not possible to make a living teaching Yoga. Conversely I have seen teachers who, while serious about their training, have not had the benefit of obtaining a formal certification standard, yet their amiable personalities and caring way with students have allowed them to become very successful in their communities. In a similar vein, there are many medical doctors who are qualified to practice yet who lack even the most basic communication savvy and so make poor decisions, despite their thorough training. It is unlikely that we would then conclude that it isn't necessary for a doctor to be properly educated in his field. Rigorous training to become a Yoga teacher is important, whether it leads to a certificate or not. It is the most reliable means we have for establishing and maintaining a standard within the profession, but it is no guarantee (just as a medical license is no guarantee) that the practitioner will be a good one.

The primary issue is whether teachers have had a sound and thorough training in the subject they wish to teach others, regardless of whether they have a piece of paper to prove it. At the very least, completion of a certification program is some measure of the seriousness and sincerity of the trainee. It is not uncommon for people to realize during the course of a program that, while they feel a commitment to their own Yoga practice, they do not want to teach. Some discover that they enjoy teaching occasional small classes in their homes but that full-time teaching is not to their liking and may even undermine their joy for the practice, the way a happy home cook may not want to work in a restaurant.

In considering any training program, I would ask whether, by attending classes with the graduates and faculty of this program, you have established that the classes are safe, skillfully sequenced, and enjoyable. It would be important to me that the physical practices be presented as part of the larger context of Yoga as a spiritual path.

There are now umbrella organizations that consider an individual's training (often obtained from many different sources) and certify these individuals according to a certain set of curricular requirements. While this is a step in the right direction, there are some major disadvantages to this approach. Obtaining two training hours from twenty different teachers, in twenty different contexts, does not equal forty hours of cumulative training with one qualified teacher. A hodgepodge of accumulated training hours can never equal consistent practice, study, and supervision with a few teachers over a long period of time. The jury is still out on whether such organizations will raise or lower standards within the Yoga profession. I hope that in the future such organizations will structure their curricular requirements in such a way as to encourage more cohesive education. On the other hand, there are many teachers who, for family reasons or because they live in a small town or community, are unable to attend long training sessions. Having a goal of completing two hundred or five hundred hours of Yoga teacher training, in whatever form one is able, will undoubtedly motivate many to further their education. At the very least, knowing that a teacher has had a minimum of two hundred hours of training is some insurance for the general public.

There are also widely respected teachers who have had little or no formal training but who have spent a lifetime in self-study and practice. Their devotion to practice and to the tradition itself is apparent in the self-discipline required to continue such study. These teachers are rarely motivated to teach for commercial reasons, and their authenticity is rewarded by devoted students. As well, many respected contemporary teachers, after studying a particular method rigorously for a number of years, develop their own unique approach, usually after deep self-inquiry and years of research and development in their classes.

For anyone considering training as a Yoga teacher, the bottom line is this: Will this course give me a sound, thorough, and safe foundation to teach the skills I wish to offer my students? Sometimes training programs offer popularity by association but do not necessarily offer sound training. You need to reflect honestly about your own intentions in pursuing your study and act accordingly.

Misapprehension is that comprehension which is taken to be correct
until more favorable conditions reveal the actual nature of the object.

THE DANGERS OF CHARISMA
AND THE PITFALLS OF FAME

The magnetism and charm of an individual can have a strong allure, especially
when there is the possibility of power by association. While there are undoubtedly teachers who back up their natural presence with substantial substance, so there are teachers whose sparkling veneer (often generated by years
of marketing machinery) is just that—a brittle patina covering an empty center. My advice to students is to deeply investigate and substantiate whether a
teacher truly has something of worth to offer. Detach yourself from the
"buzz" of working with a well-known teacher or getting caught up in the
scene of a packed Yoga class, and discern whether you are actually learning
something from this person. Are her classes thoughtfully planned, logically
sequenced, and filled with useful information, or do her classes seem more like
workouts designed to impress the crowd? Are his instructions clear, concise,
and informed by the teacher's own personal experience, or are his comments
a compilation of the latest New Age platitudes? Sometimes a teacher who at
first appears quiet and unprepossessing turns out to have great depth and wisdom. When presenting at Yoga conferences, I am often amazed at the superb
standard of teaching offered by little-known teachers (often with very small
audiences in attendance) and the embarrassingly vacuous teaching offered by
some of the most touted Yoga stars in sold-out classes. One wonders whether
such teachers have begun to believe their own marketing promotions, such is
the confidence with which they present their feeble offerings.

There will always be leaders like this, whether they are religious leaders with huge bank accounts or political leaders with corrupt connections. And there will always be gullible followers of such leaders. Whenever considering study with a teacher, whether he be well-known or not, proceed with eyes wide open and with a discerning mind. Just as it would be unwise to move in with someone after the infatuation of a first date, it can be equally unwise to offer a teacher unqualified trust and commitment before he has proven the mettle of his character. So take whatever time is necessary to thoroughly investigate a teacher before making a deeper commitment to further study. Then regularly review what you are getting from the teacher. At the end of each class, ask yourself: What did I learn today that is of value in my Yoga practice and in my life?

I am not saying that all teachers who are popular are deserving of suspicion. There are those whose years of faithful service that have been rewarded with immense popularity. Often this popularity comes after decades of relative professional obscurity and sparse financial rewards. The danger for any teacher in attaining popularity is a tendency to rest on one's laurels. One does not have to try as hard when it is assured that the registration will be full, with a waiting list, regardless of whether one practices, prepares, or plans for a teaching event.

Whether popularity has been earned by true worth or not, there are potential pitfalls to fame. When a teacher receives adoration from increasing numbers of students, it is common for these same students not to question the actions of the teacher. The more powerful a teacher becomes, the more intimidating she may be to a student and therefore the less likely a student will keep the teacher's ego in check by respectful questioning and confrontation. Such a teacher may become swept up in her own egotism and even come to believe that normal rules and laws do not apply to her. This is a classic scenario that has been repeated throughout history by leaders of all kinds. So it should not surprise us that within the Yoga tradition, especially since the transplantation of Yoga from East to West, many teachers have fallen from grace. Whenever abusive actions are rationalized and justified by a teacher's followers, we should be extremely wary. Whenever a teacher's abusive actions are covered up or denied, we should see this for what it is: complicity. Although a teacher's abusive actions are her responsibility, students also have a responsibility to themselves, to other students, and to the tradition to challenge such teachers, thereby creating a healthy environment of checks and balances. Even more important, a teacher's peers have the responsibility to challenge her abusive behavior.

One well-known teacher who carried the mantle of a Yoga lineage had for years been the subject of whispered rumors about inappropriately touching his students. His actions were—in any context, Eastern or Western—sexually indecent and illegal. If a man were to put his hand up my dress on the street, it would be called sexual assault. But somehow, within the context of a Yoga class, people have come to believe that a teacher placing his hands on a woman's genitals without her permission is justified if it is to demonstrate the action of a mudra.[2] Because of this teacher's respected standing, these reports remained largely ignored, the character of the women was questioned, and the legitimacy of their claims was doubted. Then in a teaching tour of the United States, a number of female students, unaccustomed to having a Yoga teacher place his hands on their genitals, openly challenged his behavior in a public class. I do not know how this situation was resolved, but I have noticed that this teacher hasn't toured the United States in recent times.

While going to the police or confronting a teacher publicly is not an ideal way to handle such a situation, the Yoga community has forced the issue by having few if any formal channels through which to process such cases. If this teacher's own senior students had challenged his behavior long ago and made it clear that it was unacceptable, it is unlikely it would have continued unchecked for so long. I want to be perfectly clear that responsibility always rests in the hands of the teacher, but there can be complicity within the community when students, and those who host such teachers, do not question or investigate substantiated cases of abusive behavior.

Sutra III.46

What constitutes perfection of the body?
Beauty, grace, strength, and adamantine firmness.

Medical Concerns and Making Unfair Claims

Yoga teachers, especially *hatha* Yoga teachers need to be careful in the claims they make about their work. For example, teachers should never claim to have powers they do not possess. Promising that a student's condition will improve is unethical. Communicating that you have seen others in a similar condition improve, but that you can make no promises, offers encouragement where it may be sorely needed without exploiting the vulnerability of someone in need.

Yoga teachers who are not medically qualified should not make medical diagnoses or counter a diagnosis made by a medical practitioner. A teacher should never advise a student to stop taking medication, but they may advise that the student obtain current advice from her physician or other qualified health care practitioner.

Handling medical issues can often be a sticky matter, especially when a teacher believes that a student's physical problems have not been accurately assessed. Frequently physicians with little or no knowledge of musculoskeletal problems make absolute and very discouraging statements about the prognosis of physical problems that have been shown to be helped by Yoga. Just as frequently they make blanket statements about the efficacy of Yoga practice with no knowledge of the sophistication of Yoga therapeutics or its many highly skilled teachers.[3] In this situation it is better to let the proof be in the pudding, allowing the student to come to his or her own conclusions. If there is any doubt, however, about the safety of a student beginning Yoga practice, he should gain the approval of his health practitioner first. The following list may help you in making ethical decisions for the welfare of your students:

- Prior to beginning class, always ask whether students have any injuries or health conditions that might affect their participation in your class. If you have a preregistration form for your courses, consider asking questions about health and medical conditions and any current prescriptions the student may be taking.

- Offer care and encouragement but don't promise a cure. Refrain from making a diagnosis when unqualified to do so.

- Always respect the diagnosis, treatment protocol, and medications prescribed by a qualified heath practitioner.

- If you feel out of your depth, consider referring a student to another teacher who is more experienced or has specific experience working with a particular health condition.

- Err on the side of caution: refer the student back to her health practitioner to make sure that Yoga is a safe and appropriate practice.

- Always ask the student's permission to contact the attending health practitioner to get a fuller picture of his health status.

- Let the proof be in the practice: students will draw their own conclusions when they experience improvement or resolution of a health condition.

- Request that a student working in a special-needs class, retreat, or residential training disclose any current medications he is taking and the health condition being treated by those medications. It can be argued that all students attending Yoga classes should disclose such information. In particular, pain relief and anti-inflammatory medications can mask symptoms, making it difficult to ascertain a student's safe threshold for movement. Also, those on psychiatric medications for mental illness should be screened to determine their suitability for inclusion in practices such as long meditation retreats.

In my application screening process of teacher trainees I frame it this way:

> *Do you have any physical or emotional conditions that could affect your participation in the training? An important aspect of this training is its highly experiential nature. You will be working deeply with yourself and closely with other individuals and the group as a whole. You will be presented with a range of different teaching and learning styles, some of which you may be unaccustomed to. While emotional issues can sometimes arise for some people, participants need to have experience in processing, expressing appropriately, and containing these experiences. If you are currently undergoing psychiatric or psychotherapy treatment and/or are taking psychiatric medications, you may wish to discuss attending this training with your therapist.*

- Consider asking a student to attend private sessions if her special needs cannot be met within a group class or if her condition may be made worse by attempting to keep up with the rest of the group. For some, private lessons are not possible for financial reasons. (Please see the section on Class Levels for information on class structures that may accommodate such students.)
- Maintain confidentiality about a student's health condition unless otherwise agreed.

ETHICAL INQUIRY:
STUDENT SAFETY

During a weekend workshop, the hosting teacher brought my attention to Sophia, who was having severe emotional reactions after class. I was rather surprised to discover Sophia attending a small private dinner normally reserved for coteachers, hosts, and myself. Taking me aside, the host said that Sophia seemed extremely fragile and she had invited her to the dinner as an act of support. Both Sophia and her husband had a history of drug addiction and alcohol abuse and in Sophia's case several instances of threatened self-harm. As a new mother in an unstable relationship and financially insecure, she was under considerable stress. During the dinner Sophia said privately to my coteacher, "I might as well kill myself" and made other statements that caused concern. After a brief discussion we advised the directors of the center to immediately direct Sophia to a local suicide help line. They counseled her not to be by herself for the next twenty-four hours and strongly urged her to go to a community mental health center the next day for immediate care. ▇ ▇

ETHICAL INQUIRY:
REFERRING A STUDENT
TO A MEDICAL PRACTITIONER

Katrina was a regular student who had privately expressed her anguish at having recently had an abortion. After inquiring more fully, I discovered that she was still bleeding and, while making it clear that she had my emotional support, I asked her not to attend class until her bleeding had stopped and she had the okay from her doctor to resume physical activity. Katrina resumed classes a few weeks later and all seemed well. Six months later, Katrina called me at home one evening to say she was having severe abdominal pain that was not relieved by any position. She did not divulge any further details but wanted my advice as to what she could do through Yoga to ameliorate her pain. First I expressed that, as I was not a medical doctor, I could not give her advice and that if the pain was severe she should immediately go to the emergency room at her local hospital. I later discovered that Katrina had an abdominal abscess that had become septic (a potentially life-threatening condition) caused by another abortion. I visited her in the hospital and later, when she was better, expressed my concern that she practice greater discernment in her sexual relations to prevent further harm to herself and to another. ■ ■

ETHICAL INQUIRY:
MAKING UNFOUNDED CLAIMS

During my last few years of teaching Yoga in San Francisco, during the height of the AIDS epidemic (and long before the advent of life-prolonging drugs), I noticed that the predominantly gay Castro district was being showered with glossy brochures promoting a new form of Yoga. As these new classes were going to be offered at the studio where I rented space, I decided to attend the "opening launch," in which the senior teacher of the method would give a lecture. A colleague and I showed up to the opening, joining about a hundred others, some clearly ill with AIDS.

The senior instructor, dressed in tight, revealing white pants, a shirt unbuttoned to his navel, and enormous gold chains, began his lecture with a fanfare of applause by those seated at the front. We had the distinct impression that these people (who were dressed in formal suits) had been planted in the audience to set the necessary tone of adoration. After several minutes, the speaker made an extraordinary statement: "If you practice my method, you will be healed of AIDS!" Having just completed the first-ever university course on the biology of AIDS, and having a fairly good grasp of the nature and prognosis of the disease at that time, I found this statement deeply disturbing. I had witnessed the rapid decline and death of a number of my students and Yoga colleagues. After another thirty minutes of self-aggrandizing oratory peppered with foul language, my colleague and I made for the door. Classes did indeed begin at the studio, but after only a few months the regional teacher of the method became too ill to teach. We understood that the teacher was HIV-positive, but no explanation for his departure was given. ■ ■

When to Send a Student to Another Practitioner

Whenever you as a teacher believe that a student's problems, whether they be psychological, emotional, physical, or spiritual, lie outside the domain of your expertise, it is only wise (and compassionate) to refer such a student to a more suitable and possibly more experienced practitioner, whether that be another Yoga practitioner, a doctor, a counselor, or a therapist. In working with female Yoga students with a history of sexual abuse, such as incest, if the student is in an acute stage of processing, I almost always insist that they also be working with a psychotherapist or psychiatrist who is qualified to handle sexual abuse issues and is monitoring their progress. I might also ask such a person to seek her practitioner's approval to attend a retreat, intensive, or meditation seminar because sometimes intensive work brings up unresolved issues. Such a student needs to be able to fall back on her security net of support to safely address her issues.

When a student has a serious health condition that does not seem to be improving through his Yoga practice, it is always advisable to ask the student to seek medical advice. Sometimes what can appear to be a musculoskeletal problem, such as a sore lower back, can be a serious organic or physiological condition, such as a kidney infection, tumor, or neurological condition. Whenever a student complains of pain that is not alleviated by any position, such as lying on the back or side, or is severe enough to prevent him from sleeping, it is important to advise him to seek medical advice. I recall one such student who complained of intense abdominal pain that did not shift, regardless of whether she was standing, lying down, or using a heating pad. I advised her to go to the hospital immediately, where she was diagnosed with an intestinal blockage which, if left untreated any longer, could have been very serious.

Yoga teachers should also carefully assess their own prejudices about health care, because these may cloud their judgment. If a Yoga teacher believes that all health conditions can and should be resolved through Yoga practice alone, or only with the help of natural, herbal, or alternative health modalities, he may fail to see when a condition requires allopathic medical intervention. A student with knee problems may very well require surgery, not only to alleviate current pain but also to prevent further damage to the joint. A teacher who insists that such a student solve his knee problems through Yoga may inadvertently cause further injury. Similarly if a teacher takes a strong or dogmatic position about health care, this may prevent a student from seeking necessary medical help.

We need to take students' perceptions seriously and respectfully. We also need to respect the territory of other professionals and not cross boundaries into areas where we have no training. Even if a Yoga teacher has the training to work therapeutically, it is often wiser to do so with the cooperation of the student's other health practitioners. For instance, in working with people with spinal problems, a teacher might ask the student's permission to speak with his chiropractor, orthopedist, or body worker in hopes of getting a clearer picture of how to help. Many health practitioners enthusiastically enter into such tandem work, especially when they see their clients improving through their Yoga practice.

In particular, Yoga teachers should not play pop psychologists or deliberately provoke emotionally cathartic experiences in students who may be unprepared and unable to integrate such experiences. This is particularly disturbing if the teacher is simply visiting a center and will not be there to help pick up the pieces later.

ETHICAL INQUIRY:
APPROPRIATE INTERVENTION

Douglas was teaching a seminar as a guest instructor. He put Celia into a supported Shoulderstand (Sarvangasana) with the use of a chair. The position was quite extreme and, instead of carefully supervising Celia, Douglas went on to teach the rest of the class. By the time Celia came out of the position, she stated that she felt unwell. The hosting director noticed that she was extremely pale, and when Celia suddenly went in to the bathroom, she followed Celia out of concern. She discovered Celia unconscious on the bathroom floor, blue in the face, faintly breathing. She called for help from another student who was a nurse, and when Celia felt well enough to return to the studio, the director communicated to Douglas that the woman had lost consciousness. Douglas then casually dismissed this revelation, saying, "Oh, she'll be all right". By way of help, he rifled through his bag and offered Celia an herbal drink product, which he was selling. How would you have responded to this situation if you were the director?

ETHICAL INQUIRY:
IT'S OKAY TO SAY YOU DON'T KNOW

This inquiry was contributed by a colleague.

"In a Western culture we are pretty much expected and taught to always have an answer to every question. In school we are taught to not leave any blanks on a test. It is considered better to give any answer with the possibility of it being correct rather than nothing at all. Our culture makes it shameful and not okay to not know. Does our personal practice leave enough latitude so that as teachers and as human beings we are able to simply and humbly say, 'I simply don't have the answer to that question'? Maybe it's the ethics of pride and humility, the ethics of being able to say, 'I don't know' when asked a question we don't have the answer to, instead of faking it and replying with 'I think that' or 'I guess that,' thereby contributing to cloudy and murky information, which the recipient will take as accurate because it came from a teacher. I wonder if perhaps this scenario is played out all too often in order to not risk coming across as uninformed, uneducated, or stupid.

"Some years ago I brought in a highly qualified qigong instructor to a class. Not too long into the class, someone asked her a question, to which she replied, 'I don't know.' She didn't try to pad it with questionable facts. Shortly after that, she responded to another and yet another question in the same way. At first I was a little embarrassed. Then I noticed that when she did answer a question she spoke with a confident and strong voice. I also noticed that she said 'I don't know' with a strong voice. There was neither shame nor defensiveness in her 'I don't know.' That made all the difference. At first people were taken aback by the frequency of her 'I don't know' responses, but by the end of the weekend they had a lot of respect and affection for her. She was a confident, strong, and well-educated teacher. Her honesty gave her integrity and credibility. Her example of saying 'I don't know' without embarrassment gave all of us permission to do the same. Talk about freeing up energy!"

Notice what happens to you when you are asked a question you do not know the answer to. Are you able to give an honest reply? In a similar vein, do you feel uncomfortable creating pauses within your instructions for fear that students will think you don't know something? What happens for you (and for your students) when you rest in stillness between instructions? ■ ■

SUTRA II.37

When we are firmly established in integrity, all riches present themselves freely.

Class Numbers

Whether you are a studio director organizing a workshop with a visiting teacher or a teacher offering a beginning Yoga class at a local church hall, consider what is fair and equitable in deciding limits on class numbers. Increasingly I hear distressing accounts of sincere beginners entering Yoga classes at the local gym or Yoga studio surrounded by fifty people. Although it is not impossible to teach a safe beginning class to such numbers (as many of my colleagues are required to do in university settings), when a large class size is combined with a speedy pace and inappropriately difficult practices and postures, the results can be disastrous. Frequently beginning students abandon their budding Yoga practice out of sheer frustration, or they discover, when they attend a new class elsewhere, that what they were learning was not Yoga at all but sophisticated calisthenics with Sanskrit names.

In considering class numbers, both the experience level of the students and the experience level of the teacher should be factored in. Generally when people are being introduced to a new skill, the numbers should be smaller to allow for more personal attention. When I first began teaching in my home, I worked with groups of four to ten people, which allowed me to develop important skills, such as balancing group instruction with the need to give individual attention, while still maintaining the pace of the class. Working with smaller numbers also allowed me to develop skills in identifying problems common to the group and thus helped me to refine my instructions. Later, when I began renting a studio and had greater experience in pacing a group class, I limited beginning-level classes to twenty or twenty-five students. Many beginning-level students come with preexisting health issues and complex physical problems, and because they have little or no experience in posture work, they don't know how to modify postures for their condition. Unlike intermediate students who know how to identify good pain from bad pain and know how to adapt a posture, beginners do not have this ability, and therefore they are the most vulnerable of all students. It is my preference, even with small beginners groups, to have a teaching assistant to accommodate the need for one-to-one attention throughout the class. Some Yoga traditions go as far as saying that one-to-one teaching is the only ethical way to teach Yoga. There is great merit in this stance, because it allows a teacher to address the unique circumstances and goals of each student. Even if a teacher chooses to work within a group setting, there will certainly be students who need private lessons outside of class, either on an ongoing basis or to prepare them to attend a group lesson safely. Some teachers have developed a structure of semiprivate practice sessions (limited to no larger than six people), where students practice with supervision, thereby offering the student the advantage of individual attention without the cost of a private lesson.

Theory and practice however do not always tally. The reality for many Yoga centers with high overhead costs is that class numbers may need to be higher than is ideal. Covering the costs of running a center and paying instructors a reasonable wage can be a difficult balancing act. Many of the studio directors I work with express the challenge of combining a viable business with offering teachings that have integrity. Higher class numbers however can be mitigated by a number of possible options: offering clearly designated class levels (more about this later), offering six- or eight-week courses for specific levels with no casual attendance (more about this, too), and having apprentices work as teaching assistants alongside more experienced teachers to lower the student-to-teacher ratio.

Class Numbers
for Workshops and Intensives

When hosting a visiting teacher, the airfare and accommodation costs alone can demand high registration numbers. There is a fine balance, however, between meeting the demand for such a teacher and creating a potentially poor learning environment for the students. Such teachers can often bring a trained and adept teaching assistant with them if they have advance notice, or they may know of regional teachers who would be willing to assist them to lower the student-teacher ratio. In my experience, the small extra cost of bringing an assistant, or offering scholarships to regional teachers to help, is completely offset by the raised standard of the learning environment. Having larger numbers in a workshop or teacher-training setting is not necessarily unethical if it is clear that students have a safe learning environment and the teachings they receive are of value. When higher numbers are anticipated, though, the host needs to be honest in relaying this to students to prevent an unrealistic expectation of one-on-one attention. A visiting teacher can also request that a host carefully screen participants so that the experience level of the group is cohesive. Allowing a student with little or no experience, or someone with a complicated injury, to attend a large group Yoga workshop is doing a disservice to the student, the teacher, and the rest of the group.

Students also need to be realistic about their own expectations. Senior teachers are generally in strong demand, and there will predictably be many students who wish to have access to their teachings. When you enter a large workshop setting as a student, it is best to become an "ear to the room," learning as much as you can from group instructions and from specific instructions given to other individuals. Paying close attention to the teacher's demonstrations and to the work the teacher does with another student may provide valuable insight into your own problems. Attending a large workshop with the expectation that a teacher is going to address your complicated and long-standing neck injury is unrealistic and unfair to the teacher. It is also unfair to stay after class to ask a "short question" when what is really wanted is that the teacher listen to a long case history that would require a one-on-one private lesson. Most senior teachers will do everything within their power to help individual students, but when such a teacher is leading a large group, it can be impractical to ask for more individual attention than is offered.

The host of such an event needs to ensure that the venue is large enough to comfortably accommodate everyone, and that everyone can both see and hear the teacher, even if this necessitates a teaching platform and amplification microphone. It is unfair for a host to take more people than a room can comfortably hold, and while a large attendance might be an advantage this fiscal year, people vote with their feet and often do not return to study with a teacher when they feel the group was unmanageably large. Teachers need to skillfully consider whether their teaching material can be safely offered to large numbers and adapt the practices accordingly. For instance, in a conference setting, where the numbers are often very large and yoga props scarce, I never teach Headstand (Salamba Sirsasana) or Shoulderstand (Salamba Sarvangasana) and would be reluctant to present practices such as Handstand (Adho Mukha Vrkasana). When a practice might have an unsettling effect (as can be the case with specific Yoga Nidra practices), consider whether the students will have a chance to integrate the material, as would be possible in ongoing classes or in a longer residential retreat format. In these situations, you would be made aware of a student's difficulty and have the opportunity to investigate further.

There can be a fine line between wanting to make a teacher available to the widest possible audience and plain greed; it is not hard to crunch a few numbers and realize that allowing one hundred people into a workshop will have quite a different financial outcome than allowing only fifty. And it is not necessarily unethical to do so. Senior teachers of any discipline, whether secular or sacred, are precious resources. By the time such people have attained mastery in their field, they will also have probably garnered a large and eager audience. When a teacher has reached this level of attainment, most students realize that making the teachings available to as many people as possible precludes the kind of intimate interactions with the teacher they might expect in another context. There is a quantifiable difference too between having one hundred people in an asana workshop learning Headstand (Salamba Sirasana) for the first time, and the same number of people attending a lecture or meditation practice or being guided into deep relaxation.

The bottom line that teachers and Yoga center directors must address, regardless of their circumstances, is at what point the numbers in a class setting drastically affect the ability of the teacher or center to deliver what they have promised to give: a safe learning environment in which new skills can effectively be learned.

A Word about Amplification

Initially many people have a negative reaction to a Yoga teacher using a headset microphone. This is unfortunate, because this technology can and should be used to radically improve the quality of instruction when class numbers are large. Traveling Yoga teachers who lead guest workshops, where the class numbers are generally much bigger than in an ordinary class, need to use amplification. I highly recommend that traveling Yoga teachers invest in their own equipment. I now travel with my own headset microphone to ensure a high quality of sound (the quality of rental microphones is generally very poor) and to ensure that the equipment is comfortable (rental equipment can be ungainly or unsuitable, as is the case in clip-on microphones, which are not designed for a moving speaker).

Once students get over their initial reaction to amplification, most are delighted to be able to hear all the instructions. Many have told me that this is the first Yoga workshop in which they have been able to hear all the instructions. Older students with hearing problems are especially appreciative, and for certain practices, where lying down decreases people's auditory ability, amplification is essential. Additionally, in larger rooms and in rooms with poor acoustics, a Yoga teacher only has to turn his head in one direction, or bend down to adjust a student, and half of the room misses an instruction, no matter how well he projects his voice. Hosts should also keep in mind that a guest teacher may be required to project his voice for up to six hours a day during an intensive, and in longer trainings to sustain this activity for a week or more. This places a severe demand on any voice, and it is unnecessarily exhausting. When projecting into a large room, you also can use only a limited range of expression, which I've found does not allow the kind of subtle inflection I might want to impart to an instruction during meditation or while leading Corpse Pose (Savasana). Hosts need to be aware that intensive teaching is quite a different animal from a regular hour-and-a-half class taught in a smaller room, and they should ensure that amplification is available.

SUTRA II.36

When we are firmly established in truthfulness,
action accomplishes its desired end.

ETHICAL CLASS STRUCTURES

How many university professors would be able to successfully teach their courses if students from all levels (from those with no experience to graduate students) attended the same course? Would a university lecturer attempting to cover a specific curriculum allow anyone at any time to drop in and waylay the class with questions that clearly showed their lack of prerequisite study? Imagine a professor trying to teach a course in advanced genetics to students who had not so much as attended a basic chemistry course. This is the situation that Yoga teachers face when working at many Yoga centers worldwide.

To offer sound teaching, we need to look seriously at the structure of Yoga classes. When a class is open to an endless stream of casual drop-in students, some with serious physical injuries and health conditions, we can neither honor the needs of those vulnerable students nor, as important, meet the needs of the devoted regular students who wish to progress in their practice. When classes are open to anyone of any level, and students can enter a class at any time, the students who suffer most are the ones who have made the greatest commitment. Each time a beginning student enters a public class, a teacher may be required to drop the level of the class to the lowest common denominator to maintain safety. This is one of the most commonly discussed problems in teacher-training programs, and struggling to offer a better class in a structure that is inherently unsound is like bailing water from a boat without repairing the leaking hole. To remedy this situation, I strongly believe that Yoga classes should require preregistration, with at the very least a certain number of fundamental classes required as prerequisites for any student wanting to attend an open class. There are tremendous advantages to this structure, including:

- The teacher now has the ability to build information cumulatively, having determined the skills he wishes to teach within a particular course time.

- The cohesive structure of one group of students allows the teacher to familiarize herself with the needs of those individuals. Additionally, because students are not allowed to casually drop in, the needs of those registered remain foremost.

- The students are required to make a commitment. Many centers believe this is not possible, but in my experience of running a center and changing from open classes to registered courses, the students expressed gratitude for learning discipline and being required to stay with something they knew to be beneficial. The center almost tripled its income due to the popularity of these courses.

- The teacher and the center have a guaranteed income for a particular course. Whether students then attend all the classes is their decision, while the teacher, having made the commitment, is rewarded regardless.

- The teacher is able to witness an improvement from the beginning to the end of the course. Being able to see and appreciate tangible results is essential for career satisfaction, and this experience of accomplishment is a crucial factor in career longevity.

- Centers develop strong reputations from offering sound instruction to their students. In the case of one center, word-of-mouth about the small class numbers and excellent courses allowed the center to radically reduce its advertising budget, and subsequent courses began to fill, many with waiting lists.

Such consideration for the integrity of the structure of classes should also be extended to workshops and intensives. In my own contractual requirements, I almost always request that there be no partial attendance for a weekend or weeklong intensive. I have experienced firsthand what happens, both as a teacher and as a participant in workshops, when students are allowed to enter a course midway. Frequently the material confuses such students because they have not been privy to important foundation material, and their questions interrupt the presentation of the material. There is also a certain group bond and intimacy that forms during a retreat, a container that allows people to feel safe in exploring vulnerable aspects of their integration. When a newcomer arrives, no matter how nice the person may be, the container is compromised, because trust in that individual has not been established. Unfortunately, if the teacher is not judicious about who she allows into a class and when, she may end up giving more energy and attention to the drop-ins than to the students who made the commitment to be there the whole time. It is tempting for workshop hosts to allow such partial attendance for financial reasons, but this often undermines a cohesive learning environment.

On certain occasions allowing a person to drop in to a class may be appropriate. Sometimes a longtime student who is very familiar with my work requests entry to a single class. On other occasions a student visiting from overseas or who may be in the region for only a few days asks to attend one of my ongoing Yoga classes. On other occasions, as in a retreat, I have asked the students' permission for a newcomer to visit or observe a class. Generally however I discourage drop-in attendance because even someone observing a class can cause members of a group to feel uncomfortable.

Creating and sustaining ethical class structures is one way that teachers can provide a cohesive container for their students. When a teacher isn't clear about the boundaries necessary to uphold a sound class structure, students unconsciously register this lack of a clear boundary, and predictably some test the limits. A lack of clear boundaries can manifest in chronic student lateness, students missing classes and demanding refunds, and even students leaving class early. If the teacher is the least bit unclear about her terms, or changes the terms at the least provocation, she leaves herself and her students open to a "leaky container," that is, one that cannot support powerful teaching.

Students do need to realize that Yoga teachings are a profound gift, and that teachings are not offered on their terms alone. Teachers have a right and an obligation to make their terms clear. They are entitled to make their own requirements of students and to teach contingent upon those terms. When a teacher or center fails to make its terms clear, students are given no guidance and so form their own ideas about what is permissible.

Recently, while I was on a teaching tour of the United States, a number of center directors expressed their dismay at a new phenomenon. Students are coming for the active portion of the classes only and are rolling up their mats and walking out before the quieter floor work and relaxation portion of the class at the end. It was interesting to see the varied responses to this distressing phenomenon. Some centers immediately instructed their teachers to make it clear to students that to attend a class they had to attend the whole class, and others posted signs to make this clear to the students. This sent an unequivocal message that a code of conduct existed and adherence was required to receive these teachings. Other centers simply allowed the behavior to go unchecked and hoped things would change, leaving both teachers and students in a quandary of confusion. Again the most dedicated students attending the class had their experience disrupted time and again by people leaving at whatever time suited them. This is clearly not a good way to express appreciation to a loyal community of students.

Sutra II.46

The posture of the body during the practice of contemplation and at other times, as also the posture of the mind (or attitude to life) should be firm and pleasant.

Class Levels

Both teachers and Yoga centers have a responsibility to offer clearly designated class levels with clearly defined content. Following on the previous discussion about class structure, this is unlikely to be possible when students of any level are allowed to attend any class of their choosing. Teachers need to screen participants carefully to determine an appropriate level, as new students are often incapable of determining this for themselves. Many believe that the one class they took ten years ago, or their brief experience with a television Yoga series or video, qualifies them to attend an intermediate or advanced class. More important than the actual logistics of setting up a class schedule and advertising for specific classes is that the teacher actually teaches to the level advertised. In this regard Yoga centers hiring teachers have a responsibility to ensure that teachers are working within safe parameters, especially when teaching absolute beginners. Unfortunately many teachers, especially young ones, may feel pressured to deliver a more advanced or more rigorous class than would be wise for the participants because they anticipate that this may garner them greater popularity. This is an unfortunate dilemma, with students often wanting to work at a level that is entirely unsuited to their ability, and teachers succumbing to this perceived pressure. Many center directors have privately shared with me that they have had to remove the word *beginner* from advertising brochures because it has become an affront to the Western mind to be considered a beginner at anything! The expectation of instant gratification, whether this is from the acquisition of material possessions or the acquisition of skills, is a fairly recent cultural phenomenon, one that undermines the richness of experience that comes from a long-term commitment to any endeavor. Yoga teachers and centers can either serve or challenge this cultural pathology.

While it is simply not possible for a teacher to tailor a class perfectly to meet the needs of every individual, I like to use what I call the 90 percent–10 percent rule. If 90 percent (and hopefully more) of the class seems to understand and be able to integrate the material, I sense that I'm working within a window of optimal learning for the group. There will always be people who come to a class with their own agenda, who are not ready to understand the material, who simply don't connect with the teacher personally, or for whatever reasons fall outside this optimal window. We should be concerned however when a significant percentage of the class is floundering to meet an unrealistic standard set by the teacher. When the teacher and only a few others can successfully practice what is taught (or, as is more often the case, strain to keep up and practice beyond their ability), it is likely that the class is more about stroking the teacher's ego than about serving the students. This kind of showing off can have dire consequences: students asked to do movements and practices that they have no foundation or conditioning for may become seriously injured. When an advertised class level and the actual class taught bear no resemblance to each other, then teachers and centers put vulnerable students (many of whom will feel too intimidated to adjust a practice or come out of a pose before others) at extreme risk of injury.

Teachers should not teach material that they have not yet integrated within their own practice and embodiment. We should teach what we know, and teach what we practice. When a teacher works from theory, rather than from information based on and tested through his own direct experience, the teaching is likely to be unsound. It is unlikely that the teacher will truly know how to help the student, because he has not gone through all the necessary steps to attain mastery. It would not be unethical, however, for a teacher to teach material that he has fully mastered but no longer practices. We might compare this to the ballet mistress who knows a movement from years of personal practice and is now passing on that knowledge in her later years when she can no longer do the movement. The difference here is that at some point the information was mastered.

As a teacher you need to ask yourself about your motives when you feel a pressure to teach beyond the level of the group present. Do you fear losing students to a more demanding teacher? Do you feel a need to prove your own ability and to "strut your stuff" to obtain recognition for what you have accomplished and perhaps as a vehicle for rising up a career ladder? Is there an imagined or real concern that teaching to the level present will not hold the student's attention and thereby jeopardize your standing and employment at a center? Do you need to stroke your own ego by having "advanced students" doing "advanced practices"? All these motives need to be examined. I advise young teachers, who often feel under tremendous pressure to deliver more advanced material in order to keep their jobs, that it would be better to supplement your income from some other source than to go against your own values. English critic, editor, and author Cyril Connolly said, "Better to write for yourself and have no public, than to write for the public and have no self." This is good advice for Yoga teachers. I do believe that ethical teaching is eventually rewarded by strong and devoted students, and a teacher is more likely to maintain the integrity of her work if she does not feel under financial pressure to make her livelihood solely from teaching.

As you can see, the issues of charisma, ambition, and fame and the issue of ethical class structures and levels are intimately and somewhat messily related. Whenever a teacher or center is under strong pressure to meet high overhead costs, there can be an equal temptation to lower standards so that the bottom line is determined by financial concerns alone. Similarly when a teacher, especially a teacher trying to establish his career, is pressured to make a livelihood solely from teaching, there can be the temptation to teach in a way that undermines essential values. For teachers, I advise having dual careers, at least in the beginning. Having some other way of making a living allows you to feel less pressured and thereby removes the temptation to lower your teaching standards.

ETHICAL INQUIRY:
A CLASS TO SUIT THE CONDITION

Clarise came to me after a serious car accident in which the vehicle had rolled, leaving her with a broken scapula and ribs and a sense of fragility about her physical capacity. After receiving medical treatment, she was still unable to lift one of her arms above shoulder height, which, she was told, was "perfectly normal." Not satisfied with the limitations of such a diagnosis (which, it is important to point out, was her conclusion, not mine), she came for an initial screening to attend a special-needs Yoga course. It was determined during this private session that a group class would jeopardize her safety, so she began attending a weekly special-needs Yoga class, designed to accommodate four to eight students, with two circulating teachers. The classes were designed around simple movements and postures and were conducted at a very slow and gentle pace that could easily accommodate the stops and starts resulting from the need for one-on-one individual alterations and adaptations. Because all the students required such attention, they were empathetic to such digressions.

After many weeks of steady progress, and now able to lift both arms triumphantly over her head, Clarise graduated to a group class. Over the years she began attending retreats and intensives and deepening her understanding of Yoga. For many years after her initial attendance at the special-needs class, Clarise expressed her appreciation for the work, stating that "there was no way I would have been able to attend any normal Yoga class after my injury." Clarise's story should give us pause to consider how we might accommodate individuals who lie outside the parameters of normal class structures. Consider whether there is a need for such a Yoga class at your center. ■ ■

ETHICAL INQUIRY:
SUBSTITUTE TEACHERS.

This inquiry was contributed by a colleague.

"A couple of years ago, a Yoga teacher who was newly qualified took over one of my morning classes. All the students were women between fifty-five and seventy years of age and needed gentle movement. The new teacher apparently was not able to adjust her teaching style to the requirements of the students. It was only by chance that I met one of the women a few months later, and she told me that the new teacher had made them do a seated forward bend and went around physically pushing her weight down on the students to get them 'further' into the position. From what I was told, none of the students had refused or complained. By the time I was told, the new teacher had left the area and I had no way of contacting her."

Do you have a policy about substitute teachers and a protocol for communicating the needs of the groups they will be leading? Consider ways of determining the best way to hand over a class to another teacher, whether for one class or as a permanent arrangement. ■ ■

Sutra II.36

One who shows a high degree of right communication, will not fail in his actions.

How We Communicate with Students

Yoga teachers communicate with their students in many ways. While one teacher may prefer to work exclusively with spoken instructions, another may use physical touch and adjustment as a major part of her teaching repertoire. Most Yoga instructors combine demonstration (both by the teacher and with students as models), spoken instructions, and physical adjustments. All modes of communication demand sensitivity toward the student's experience. In the following sections we explore how to demonstrate respect for the student's process.

First, however, a brief note about authority. A teacher is a teacher because he commands a greater depth and breadth of knowledge of a subject than a student. However, there is always more for the teacher to know and other points of view that are valid. Students can and do contribute their own knowledge to the teacher's information base and to the other students. Authority in a subject should not be confused with an authoritarian attitude, in which the teacher becomes fused or solidified around the identity of "one who knows." This kind of authority is almost always accompanied by a dismissive attitude toward a student's perceptions and discoveries, as well as defensiveness when challenged by any question or conclusion that does not tally with that of the teacher. Students gain confidence when led by teachers who deserve authority. Such teachers never need to demand respect because it has been earned through the quality of their work. When a teacher takes an authoritarian position, the energy invested in presenting a facade of certainty tends to eclipse the more important messages that may be communicated in teaching. Authority that is engendered through authentic and skillful teaching never requires an arrogant stance because the students have granted the authority. A teacher's authority is transmitted through all the forms of communication used, whether demonstration, words, or touch.

Sutra II.47

[Asanas] are mastered when all effort is relaxed and the mind is absorbed in the infinite.

Adjustments and Touching

Depending on the Yoga tradition, style, or method, and also the personal and professional predilections of the teacher, physical touch may be an integral part of the teaching method. When used correctly—that is, with sensitivity and respect—touch can be an invaluable teaching tool, especially for those students who learn primarily through their kinesthetic sense. Throughout the years, I have progressed from never asking permission to touch students, to asking only if it was an intimate part of the body, to recently making it a practice to always ask permission before touching a student. At first I was reluctant to adopt this practice because I felt that it would obstruct the flow of my classes. However, to my surprise, asking permission, such as "May I touch you? or "May I use touch to suggest another way of working?" often accompanied by "Would you be interested in trying something different?" has resulted in a number of unexpected pluses:

- The creation of a "pause" during which both the teacher and student are allowed to choose whether they wish to touch or be touched, and whether they are willing to try something new.
- The rallying of both the teacher's and the student's full awareness to the process. Rather than being taken by surprise, the student can ready himself to be receptive to this information. In the case of the teacher, the pause may allow her to act more sensitively and deductively rather than making habitual or thoughtless adjustments.
- The acknowledgment that a student's mere presence in class does not constitute permission to touch her.
- The recognition on the part of the student that she has a responsibility to maintain whatever boundaries are necessary for her to feel safe and respected. In this teacher–student paradigm, the mode of communication is shared.
- The acceptance that there are times when a student, for whatever reason, does not want to be touched.

A teacher should never continue to touch a student if the student has expressly asked him to stop. This is particularly important when the teacher is helping a student improve her range of motion in a posture. Some horrific injuries have been incurred within our profession, most of which could have been prevented had the teacher been working within a horizontal mode of communication rather than an authoritarian or dictatorial vertical mode. When a teacher stops listening with her hands and works with a process of assumption rather than deduction, touch will rarely be effective and can be extremely injurious. These injuries might also be prevented if students realize that they have the right (and to some degree the obligation) to tell the teacher when an adjustment is too much, too painful, or inappropriate.

Also, however difficult it may be, it is important for the student to report back to the teacher if she has been injured. Such a report is unlikely to occur however if the teacher has taken the attitude that he is beyond reproach. This can have far-reaching consequences for both student and teacher. The teacher is unlikely to learn about his mistakes. When a student feels unable to approach the teacher directly, she will likely speak about the incident to other people, which can undermine a teacher's reputation. This however should not be the foremost reason for a teacher being open to feedback. The willingness to consider that a mistake was made, to make amends to the student if possible, to learn from the mistake, and to prevent such an occurrence from happening again are not likely to happen if the student is afraid of giving feedback. Learning from such mistakes can considerably expand a teacher's field of knowledge and thus contribute to sounder teaching in the future.

Students are generally forgiving and are willing to work with a teacher to heal an injury sustained in class. Often minor injuries are not caused by the teacher but are the result of either a preexisting condition or the student trying something for the first time, such as going up into a Handstand (Adho Muhka Vrkasana) and falling. Both student and teacher can discuss the possible cause of the injury, and the student can be made aware that he holds a responsibility to make decisions that involve risk.

Sutra II.36

When there is firm grounding in the perception of what is, or of truth, it is seen that an action and reaction, seed and its fruits, or cause and result are related to each other; and the clear vision of intelligence becomes directly aware of this relationship. (Or, one's words are fruitful.)

 ## The Power of Words

As important as the touch that we use (or don't use) in our interactions with others are the words we choose and the manner in which they are delivered. The meaning of a word can be powerfully altered by the volume and the tone of voice used in its delivery. Most important, we should keep in mind that words that might otherwise have a neutral meaning can be amplified to stunning proportions in the student's mind by their having been spoken by someone important to her.

The radical way in which a student can receive a teacher's words was underscored for me during a recent Yoga teacher training. In this part of the training, the teacher trainees were to instruct each other in small groups, and faculty were to sit in on each group and give feedback about the instruction. I noticed that many trainees froze and faltered the moment they became aware that I was observing their classes. Even when I delivered positive feedback to one trainee, it could have a devastating effect on another if she felt that the feedback she received was not equally glowing. During this most vulnerable part of the training, I realized that almost any comments on my part were bound to be amplified in the student's mind a hundredfold. Therefore I decided not to be present in the early sessions and had the teaching assistants sit in on them. They were instructed to wait until all the trainee's peers had given their feedback and not to add anything verbally unless there was something crucial missing. Not surprisingly, constructive critique offered by their peers was received with little affront or upset. This experience heightened my awareness of how even the most positive comment in the wrong context might leave a student feeling discouraged. We might consider then how the subtlest hint of sarcasm or harshness in tone of voice could be destructive to a fragile student.

But speak we must! It is important that our language reflect the kind of healthy relationship with self we wish to facilitate in the other. When a teacher yells instructions, or uses words that evoke a punitive relationship with the self, he is setting up a violent model for the student's own internal dialogue. Many years ago I attended a class at a Yoga conference with a teacher whose language seemed more suited for a military academy. She coarsely instructed us to "cut" our muscles to the bone, "push" ourselves to the limit, and finally advised us to "shove" ourselves up against the wall in a Handstand (Adho Mukha Vrksasana). This instruction to "shove" myself left me so disconcerted that I quietly rolled up my mat, excused myself with a terrible headache, and for the first time in what must have been thousands of classes, I left. I had spent too many years generating a healthy relationship with myself to want to shove myself anywhere!

More subtle is the way in which language, by its very limitations, can separate the person from the action, increasing rather than decreasing a sense of dissociation from the body. Notice the subtle differences in these instructions:

"Stretch your muscles to the limit." Or, "Invite your muscles to open."

"Push with the arm to twist the spine further." Or, "Keep the arm stable and as you exhale feel for the moment when the spine is ready to rotate."

"Breathe in for four counts." Or, "Allow the breath to enter for four counts."

Notice that in the first instruction, there is someone doing something to somebody, thereby setting up a separation between mind and body. In the second instruction, the action originates from the inside, and the actor and the action are unified. Also notice that the second instruction in each case asks the student to make an internal inquiry rather than simply obey a command.

Through careful use of language, we can invite the student to access her own internal reference point and to encourage her independence. The teacher's commitment to facilitate this independence is part of the ethos at the heart of Yoga.

Finally there is one word noticeably missing from many Yoga teachers' vocabulary: sorry. When we make a mistake, when we speak impatiently or more harshly than we intended, it can be a powerful moment for the teacher to apologize and for the student to receive that apology. When a teacher apologizes, it is an act of respect for the student. It is also a means of expressing not only our regret but also that we hold ourselves to the same standard of behavior that we expect from our students. Admitting a mistake is a way for a Yoga teacher to express his honesty with where he is in his journey. It is also a way to prevent unnecessary hurt and future resentment. It's a simple word, and while it can take great humility to say it, this magical utterance can be healing for both teacher and student.

Sutra ii.30

Yama comprises:
1. Consideration towards all living things, especially those who are innocent, in difficulty, or worse off than we are.
2. Right communications through speech, writings, gesture, and action.
3. Non-covetousness or the ability to resist a desire for that which does not belong to us.
4. Moderation in all our actions.
5. Non-greediness or the ability to accept only what is appropriate.

Codes of Etiquette

Those that question the impact that one individual can make in the world have never been in bed with a flea! Such is the disruptive influence that even one student can have on the entire learning experience of a group. We have all been in retreats, workshops, and classes where a single student hogs the teacher's attention, badgers the teacher with endless and often inappropriate questions, and wastes class time by "thinking out loud" with what turn out to be not questions at all but vague personal reflections. Other students bend every teaching situation toward their own agenda, often when it is completely irrelevant to the material being taught and the needs and interests of the group. There is no situation that so clearly requires the teacher to take the responsibility of leadership.

It is the teacher's responsibility to ensure that the most people in a group receive the teachings. When an individual or several individuals are actively interfering with the ability of others to learn, the teacher needs to rectify the situation. Frequently such a situation arises because the teacher did not establish a clear code of conduct from the start. The advantage of making a code of conduct explicit at the beginning of a course, retreat, or intensive is that the teacher can address the whole group rather than being put in the awkward position of confronting a single individual.

Preliminary to any course, I ask my students to make the agreements listed below. Out of respect for them, I explain why I am asking for these agreements, and at the end of each suggestion I check that everyone in the group understands the agreement and is willing to abide by it. I've found that taking this short time to establish basic ground rules totally transforms the workings of the teaching environment. Then later, if people are forgetting to abide by these agreements, I'll say, "Remember our agreements!" and reiterate whatever the agreement is, such as "Please don't speak when I am speaking." I'll also explain the reason for the agreement: "Repeating instructions is draining for me and for everyone. It prevents us all from doing more meaningful work." Here are some suggestions that may help you transform your learning environment:

Promptness:

Request that your students arrive promptly, preferably five to ten minutes early, in order to settle in and be ready to start by class time. In my own courses I expressly ask late students not to enter the class during the opening chant but to wait until it is finished. Once they do enter, I request that they take a place in the back of the room rather than disrupt the class by having other people move. Further I make it clear, even in a beginning-level course, that if a student is more than ten minutes late she cannot attend that class. This is not only for reasons of safety but is my expression of respect to those students who would be disrupted. I also make it clear that the most important introductory or thematic information will be presented at the beginning, and to miss that is to miss the whole gist of the class. It goes without saying that the teacher must model this behavior by being at her teaching engagement with enough time to start with equanimity.

Honoring Perceptions:

One of the most important agreements I make with my students is a request that they listen to their own inner perceptions and, more important, that they be loyal to the promptings of those perceptions. What this means to me in an asana class is that every student has a responsibility to listen to the needs of his or her individual body, mind, and emotions. In the practice of asana, honoring one's perceptions translates to many things, including adjusting a posture to accommodate an injury or health condition, coming out of a posture when you have reached your threshold and to stay longer would cause strain, asking for an alternative practice, and deciding that a certain practice is unsuitable. I give my students explicit permission to adapt the practice in such a way that they are able to honor their individual needs. I have found that it is crucial that students be given this kind of explicit permission, because most Yoga students I have worked with do not understand that they have the right and the responsibility to practice self-care. Often at the beginning of a workshop or retreat I can feel a palpable shift of relief in the room and a letting go of fear as students, some for the first time, give themselves permission to honor their own insight.

Questions:

Request that your students first internalize their questions by assessing and formulating the question intelligently. I also ask students who ask lots of questions to predetermine whether they have a true question or whether they simply want to vocalize something they already know. Such students often have other boundary issues, and by insisting that they contain their questions they learn to let their internal inquiry process gestate and mature. I also ask students to consider whether a question is relevant to the material being presented at that moment. By entertaining questions that veer away from the topic, a teacher ends up not covering the material he agreed to cover. The student may be asked to determine whether the question is of such a personal and individual nature that it would not be relevant either to the material or to the group at large. If so, I give them the opportunity to ask the question after the class is finished.

The teacher might also request that students be sitting up when they ask a question. While it may be okay for students to recline during a discussion if their backs are tired, or if they feel unwell, I still request that they make the effort to sit up if they are going to ask a question. There are times when I am also tired or unwell, yet the students certainly expect me to maintain my demeanor throughout class. I tell my students, especially those that are receiving teacher training, to "Expect from yourself what you expect of me. Hold yourself to the same standard." To demonstrate the importance of this, I casually recline back on my elbows, legs askew, and ask them how it feels to have their teacher conducting class in a reclining position. I ask them how they would feel if I were sipping coffee and nibbling on a croissant while answering their questions. When you use humor, students realize that they would find it hard to take the teacher seriously, or they might feel that the teacher is not respecting them. I also ask them to notice their level of presence when they are reclining. In the same way that they wish to be respected by the teacher sitting up and giving them full attention, they must also reflect this back to the teacher in order to be taken seriously and as a sign of respect.

Focus:

A teacher may request that students enter a studio silently out of respect for those who are attempting to change frames to begin their practice. Entering a room silently is also a great way to change gears from the extroversion of everyday life to the introversion required for Yoga practice. Additionally, when they have completed partner work, I ask students to maintain silence to allow others to complete their work undisturbed. During intensives I also request that, when students leave class to go to the bathroom, they continue to maintain silence as a way of holding their focus. (Frequently the whole class can hear a couple of students conversing on the way back to the teaching room, and it is rarely the kind of conversation we wish to be privy to.) Asking that students hold the focus is a way of communicating that they also have a responsibility for maintaining a container of concentration and that it is not only the teacher's responsibility.

Leaving Class:

If a student needs to leave class for any reason, she must alert the teacher that she is doing so. Sometimes a student may merely have a headache, or she may be so emotionally upset that she feels she can no longer be in a group. Telling the teacher allows the teacher to follow through if necessary and in many cases relieves the group of worry about the other. In retreats the group bond can be intense, and it is remarkable how the departure of one person can cause alarm in the other participants for the duration of the class. Also, if a student is unwell, she may require assistance, which was the case recently at a retreat when a student became nauseous and later discovered she had a mild case of heat stroke. Having an assistant look after her and get a resident nurse to help was imperative.

Since making an explicit code of etiquette and conduct for students coming to intensives, retreats, and trainings, I have seen a radical improvement in the quality of the teaching environment. Initially some students are taken aback by these suggestions, often because they have been studying at a center with a laissez-faire attitude. Inevitably, usually within a few days, everyone notices how much more we are accomplishing. When I have had to address the behavior of a few individuals, I am often surprised at how many other students come up after class and thank me for addressing the situation because it was driving them crazy too!

I recall when I first, and somewhat awkwardly, introduced a code of etiquette at the beginning of a teacher training. Having never done it before, I was nervous about the students' response, and sure enough many seemed mildly annoyed. The very next day a woman came to class who had arrived late the previous evening and had not heard my little talk on etiquette. She spent the first class blatantly breaking every agreement the rest of the group had made, and I watched as people's eyes widened with recognition—this is what happens when there are no clear agreements!—because they realized how much one person can affect the whole learning environment. With some excitement, the group related at the end of the class that they now realized how important these agreements were for everyone, and a number of students arranged to pass on the code to the newcomer. Since those first awkward beginnings, I have put my reluctance aside, and I hope that you, the reader, will too.

Even after making a code of etiquette clear, as a means of creating a safe and sacred environment where people can study intensively, there will always be individuals who push the boundaries. A first tack to take is to reiterate the specific point of conduct to the whole group, in hopes that the individual will recognize her behavior and adapt accordingly. Then I wait to see whether or not there is a change within the class or, in an intensive, whether there is a change over the course of the day. If not, and if I have a teaching assistant, I will ask her to address the issue with the student prior to class or after class. I have found that the advantage of this is that it can be less embarrassing for the student. It is not always possible for a teacher to have an assistant, in which case the teacher needs to speak privately with the student after the class so she will not suffer any public discomfort or humiliation. There are instances when an issue needs to be addressed in front of the group, but I usually do this only as a last resort, when someone has repeatedly ignored a request. It's important to be clear that we do this not to put down the individual; we do it to ensure the very best learning environment for everyone. It can also be enormously important for a student to have clear boundaries established and maintained.

An example of this was an individual attending a long training who consistently held up the group with his lateness. Long after all fifty other people were sitting and ready to begin a guided meditation, this person would walk in late, zip and unzip bags, rustle paper, and so on. One day I found myself becoming intensely irritated and could only imagine how others felt. So the next day, when this student yet again walked in late and began his noisy ritual, an assistant told him that he was too late for class and to please leave. Further she explained that if he wished to attend class, he must come on time. Not surprisingly, given the strength of the pattern, the student later spent hours trying to justify his need to be late, but the assistant admirably held her ground, listened to the reasons, and repeated that if he wanted to take the class, he needed to be there on time. After all, she reasoned, the student was living on site! At this point, all lateness ceased, and there was a significant change of attitude within the student, as well as what can only be described as a rather remarkable transformation. My coteacher and assistant also remarked on this change.

When the student had first arrived, I noticed within myself an aversion to him; even his facial expression seemed ugly to me. In the days that followed, I observed that his transgression of boundaries played itself out in many ways: in inappropriate comments, social ineptness, and attempts to get attention that resulted in alienating others. After we enforced the boundaries with him, it was as if he realized, perhaps for the first time in his life, that he could be seen and appreciated by others by respecting them rather than offending them. My aversion to him abated, and I also noticed that the other attendees, who had backed away from what they perceived to be an obnoxious individual, became more open and friendly toward him. This individual had been outraged by our requests and so angry for days that he refused to even return a smile. I had to trust that what we had done collectively (myself, the coteacher, assistants, and to some degree the rest of the group in keeping their agreements) was the right thing to do. I wasn't going to back down just because he was having a tantrum. As a teacher, whenever you challenge a student's longstanding pattern, you need to be prepared for these kinds of reactions, and you need to have the resolve to not back down in the face of those reactions. When you make a decision and then back down, you create confusion and only reinforce the old behavior.

When a student frequently transgresses what can be considered normal, respectful, and courteous behavior within a class setting, you can bet that this is also the way she operates in other areas of her life. By addressing the behavior within the context of a Yoga lesson, we offer her the opportunity to change that behavior, not only in class but in all aspects of her life. This can have far-reaching positive consequences.

Undoubtedly addressing such behavior can be awkward, but you can make the situation easier for yourself by developing detachment from the personal perspective of the behavior (however irritating it may be) and seeing the situation from the larger perspective of a whole life. This allows you to say something difficult, not out of a desire to be punitive but with the clear desire to offer the person a more liberating alternative behavior to the one they know.

ETHICAL INQUIRY:
SETTING SAFE PARAMETERS

An apprentice teacher at a Yoga studio reported to me that one of her students was refusing to follow her instructions. The student had a chronic back problem and refused to modify her Sun Salutation (Surya Namaskar) practice by stepping back into a lunge rather than jumping back, as is done in more advanced practice. After she told me the story, I asked her, "What did you do when she ignored your repeated requests?" "I didn't do anything," the teacher replied. "I figured it was her call." A few weeks later, a report came back to the teacher from a local sports medicine clinic. The student had gone there for treatment for her back, declaring that she was injured doing Yoga at that particular yoga studio.

While a teacher generally makes every effort not to publicly embarrass a student, when it is a matter of safety, the matter must be addressed immediately. Such students are a liability to a center, and I would not be concerned if they subsequently chose to go elsewhere. In my discussions with the beginning teacher, I suggested these options:

- Politely repeat your request, stating that "While you are free to practice however you like at home, for your safety, when you are in my class I ask that you follow my instructions."
- If a student blatantly ignores a request, a teacher has little alternative but to offer this ultimatum: "Please stop what you are doing. I will give you two choices. You may either respect the instructions given or leave the class."

Do you have a clear protocol that you follow (or, if you are a studio director, a clear protocol for your teachers) to deal with students who do not respect instructions that are intended for their safety (to modify a posture with a block, chair or other prop or to not practice a pose that is deemed unsafe)? ■ ■

Creative Ways to Communicate Your Code

It was not where I expected to learn about Yoga studio etiquette, but there it was, right in front of me as I sat on the toilet: a friendly list of helpful hints, posted on the wall where it couldn't be missed. In the course of the day, over a number of brief visits to the bathroom, I worked my way through the entire list, and I had a very good idea of what this studio expected from me as a student. Later my colleague Taffy Frost, who runs the Yoga Tree in Seattle, and who was hosting my teaching visit, told me that all new students are given a copy of this list before their first class. If you run a studio, or even if you are an independent contractor, consider making your own list that you can send to preregistered students, give out during the first class, or post throughout your teaching space. Taffy's list is not exhaustive, but it's a great example of how we can share information about living the yogic precepts in a very accessible way. Here it is.

WELCOME TO THE YOGA TREE

A few things you should know to enhance your learning and practice of Yoga. We're glad you're here. Thanks!

Please:

- Remove shoes at the door, we practice in our bare feet.

- Never bring your cell phone into the studio, leave it in your car.

- Come to practice with an empty stomach (unless a specific condition prevents this).

- Keep water bottles off the floor (we take extra special care of our floors and spilled water doesn't help). If needed, keep water bottles off to the side and take a sip when needed.

- Be early to class. Entering class constantly late is very disruptive and disrespectful to others. If you do arrive a few minutes late, take a breath, and quietly sit at the entrance until eyes are open and movement or talking has begun. At that point, unroll your mat and enter as slowly and quietly as you can.

- Bring your own mat, it's more hygienic. We do have rental mats for $1.

- Wear comfortable exercise clothing.

- Ask questions about anything that is not clear to you. You may ask during class when appropriate or after class.

- Refrain from wearing perfume, cologne, or strong essential oils.

- If you have a health issue (illness, injury, or medical condition), please notify your instructor before class. Not every pose is appropriate for everyone.

- Let go of the competitive mind-set. Yoga is noncompetitive. It is not just a work-out, it is not just techniques for relaxation, and it is not just cross-training. It is a spiritual practice that makes the body stronger, more flexible, and generally much healthier. The purpose is to calm the mind, open the heart, and stimulate our spiritual evolution.

- Be kind and loving to yourself by accepting where you are. It is okay to come out of a pose before the teacher says to. Yoga is not "gutting it out" or "no pain, no gain." To the contrary, the body will respond beautifully when you show it kindness, acceptance, and love. Rest sometimes. Do what you can, with what you have, with where you are.

- No experience or flexibility is required to practice Yoga. Yoga is for everyone.

- Stay for the entire class. If you need to leave early, tell the teacher beforehand and exit before final relaxation.

- Finally, most classes finish with the gesture and saying Namaste. This means: I honor the place in you in which the entire universe dwells. I honor the place in you in which is of love, of truth, of light, and of peace. When you are in that place in you and I am in that place in me, we are one.

Namaste

Two similar objects appear differently, depending upon
the different mental states of the observer.

BOUNDARIES

In part 1 we discussed boundaries as they pertain to the teacher–student relationship. In this section let's look at some of the other ways that healthy
boundaries can support the fullest expression of clarity between teacher and
student.

As teachers we model healthful boundaries for our students through our
own behavior. Therefore as a teacher you need to be very clear about what you
have agreed to give and what you are unable (or do not want) to give. This is
no more clearly demonstrated than beginning and ending the class on time. It
is common for students, sometimes many students, to corral teachers after
class, keeping them up to an hour beyond the stated end of class time. When I
give a longer intensive or teacher training, I explain to the students that I do
not wish to be disturbed before class, so that I can concentrate on preparing
myself for class. I also make it clear that tea and meal breaks are as necessary
for the teacher as for the students, and that even a few questions after a class
can prevent a teacher from getting necessary replenishment. I explain this further by saying that it is my heartfelt desire to be as prepared, focused, and generous as I can within the boundaries of the class time and that being disturbed
on my break time leaves me unable to give fully during class. Paradoxically
when I request and uphold these conditions, I feel an overflowing generosity
(and the energy level to follow through on the those generous impulses),
which manifests in concentrated teaching. When I don't uphold these conditions, I begin to feel defensive and even resentful of students' demands.

You may request that students ask whether you are able to answer a question or concern before they pose the question, especially if it is right before or

right after a class. This gives you the chance to decide whether you have the energy or desire to answer a question or concern, whether it requires a specific appointment to answer the question, or whether the question could only be effectively addressed in a private lesson. By requesting that the student ask if you are available to answer a question, they become conscious of the extra time and energy they are asking from you. In that moment you are also being compassionate to yourself by recognizing your physical, emotional, or psychological limits. You may also want to consider the context of the request: in a short workshop, you may feel more able to extend the teaching beyond the class time; in a longer intensive, this might not be feasible.

Another strategy that can work well in longer retreats and intensives is to ask students to write down any urgent questions they have not had answered within the class and to place them in a box. Each day I go through the notes and try to contact each individual. Often a question will be answered in a future session, in which case I will ask the student if they would like to be the model for that session (thereby getting a "mini private lesson" to deal with their issue). At other times, one of my assistants will be assigned to work with an individual, or I will answer the question within a group class as soon as is possible. Having people write down questions not only requires that the student become clear about their inquiry, it also gives the teacher a little time to reflect on the question and how best to answer it.

I have heard of students who show up an hour early for a class and in effect obtain a private lesson. I have had students who consistently arrive late and then want to keep me after class with their concerns. When the teacher has not agreed to offer this time, the student is taking something that was not freely given. The precept of not-stealing (asteya) extends beyond the grosser manifestations of stealing, such as shoplifting. It applies anytime we take something that was not freely or explicitly offered. When someone calling on the phone first says, "Do you have a moment to speak right now?" he is checking whether you can and want to give your time and energy. The teacher's ability to establish and maintain a healthy boundary is crucial, not only for the teacher's welfare but also for helping students establish their own healthy boundaries.

In my discussions with close colleagues, I have learned that an inability to create, sustain, and if necessary defend clear boundaries is a major cause of exhaustion, illness, and career burnout. Often teachers feel guilty that they have human limits—physical, emotional, and psychic limits. Many teachers find it hard to accept that their energy is limited, and that they cannot give endlessly without consequences. A teacher may also have an unexamined belief that "being spiritual" is about boundless (boundary-less) generosity. When a teacher cannot accept her own limits, she unconsciously creates a leaky boundary, which will be just as unconsciously perceived by students and will be challenged. Many of my teacher trainees have expressed that watching me model clear boundaries has given them permission to honor their own boundaries. This is the compassion that we can extend to ourselves and thereby to others.

ETHICAL INQUIRY: THE NEEDY STUDENT

Denise was a very fragile student who seemed to have an unquenchable need for personal attention. She also seemed to fear not getting information, and she needed a lot of reassurance in class that she was on track. These needs manifested in her attempts to keep me after class with what felt like endless questions. After a particular class, in which I can honestly say she received more personal attention than any other participant, she sat close to me and asked even more questions once the class had finished. I had had time to consider Denise outside class and noticed I was closing down toward her, as were the other students. I asked her if she would sit farther away from me, and told her I was feeling frightened by her demands. I expressed that no matter how much I gave her it did not seem to be enough, and that the questions she wanted me to answer were questions only she could answer herself. I understood that my fear arose from my inability to meet her needs. I asked if she would she be willing, in the next few days, to internalize her questions and trust her own process of inquiry. I also expressed my desire to remain open toward her, and for her to develop greater independence and confidence, and that continuing her habitual behavior was unlikely to result in either consequence. Although these were difficult sentiments to express, Denise received them well, and in the ensuing days she made a rather remarkable transformation. I felt myself opening to her again, and I could lower my defenses (previously needed to uphold a fallen boundary) and use my energies instead to help her through clear teaching. ▧ ▧

ETHICAL INQUIRY:
OPENING BOUNDARIES

This inquiry was contributed by a colleague.

"I teach in my home, and prior to a class I like to do a brief asana practice and sitting meditation before the students arrive. One of my students is very ill with cancer, and she noticed that I was sitting in meditation before the class. She told me that she finds the atmosphere in my home very calm, that just being in my home is healing for her. One day she asked whether it would be okay to come and sit with me before class. This student doesn't ask any questions or disrupt my practice, and she finds that fifteen minutes of sitting together particularly healing for her, so I have agreed to let her come early.

"At the end of the class I like to build community, so I offer my small group hot tea and a little snack when the class ends at 9 o'clock. The women really enjoy this time together and have generously started to bring snack offerings, but lately they have been staying as late as 10:30. So I think I will have to find a diplomatic way to communicate that the tea and snack time must finish by 9:30."

This teacher's story is a good example of someone who is using an internal locus for making ethical decisions. Making herself more available for her student with cancer feels right to her, but she also realizes that when her students stay too late this interferes with her own need for rest. As with all other ethical considerations, an internal locus makes decision-making a flexible process. ▪ ▪

Starting and Finishing on Time

While few Yoga teachers make it a habit to arrive late for their classes, it can be equally disrespectful to continue a class long after the stated finish time. Finishing on time has not always been my forte, and I have sometimes justified going overtime as an expression of generosity. Who wouldn't be grateful for that?, I thought. But recently, attending a different kind of course (as a student), I experienced firsthand how exasperating and sometimes exhausting it can be to have a teacher continue past the stated finish time. Students are then put in the awkward position of either leaving before the teacher has finished (and feeling embarrassed at the unintended slight), or staying and pushing themselves beyond their limits in terms of concentration, or making them late for other commitments. The student can also feel that their agreement to be attentive and focused to the teacher's instructions during the agreed-upon class time has been broken. You can have the feeling in such a situation that you are being held hostage against your wishes. At one particular evening lecture, which went ninety minutes over the stated finish time to the outrageous hour of 10:30 P.M., I could only imagine that the speaker was using this captive audience to download what no one in private conversation would endure. She spoke almost nonstop for two and a half hours!

If you are in the habit of going overtime, you may need to look carefully at pacing the class, change the class structure, or simply attempt to cover less material within the class time. At the very least, if you see that you will need to go overtime, it is respectful to ask permission of the class.

Sutra II.37

Through the devoted practice of not taking things, the greatest treasures are made manifest.

The Ethics of Money

Money is an exchange of energy. Given this it is important for both parties to come away from any transaction with the sense that, value for value, the exchange has been fair and equitable. Some spiritual traditions hold that asking money for what are in essence priceless teachings is unethical in any situation, but these traditions usually exist within cultures that offer those in spiritual life the financial support to live modestly but comfortably. While such teachers may not ask for money to teach meditation or offer initiations, they may very well receive money and support from the lay community. In our Western culture, recognition of the value of spiritual teaching by the larger society is often missing, so teachers have few means to secure a livelihood unless they ask for financial compensation for their work. Even the practice of giving a donation (*dana*) can leave many Westerners confused, with some leaving less money for a two-hour discourse than they would pay for a cup of coffee and a muffin.

This confusion may be related to the Western perception that money is the primary means of exchange (rather than energy in the form of labor, food, or service), and that something that is priced cheaply or free is of little or no worth. What is often missing in this equation is the imagination to realize a consequence beyond the immediate. For example, the person who walks out of a dharma talk or lecture without donating anything may not realize that this omission may make it hard for the teacher to pay her rent, let alone continue her studies. In tightly knit communities, people understand that artists and spiritual teachers are assets to the community, that they must be supported, and that to not do so is to risk no longer having these assets. The only way that gifted practitioners of anything, whether they be cellists or poets, gymnasts or writers, can study and practice full-time is if they have the financial wherewithal to support themselves. Just as it would be difficult for an Olympic runner to reach a high standard of fitness if he were working a forty-hour week, professional Yoga teachers cannot give what is necessary to their work, whether it be ongoing self-practice and education or archiving their work in written or visual material, if they need to work another full-time job.

Additionally Westerners in particular seem to have convoluted ideas about it "not being spiritual" to talk about or be clear about financial matters (such as written contracts) or to insist that people make good on their financial agreements. I would contend that this is an incorrect understanding of what it means to be spiritual. Conducting one's business clearly and fairly is one of the highest spiritual practices, because it engenders actively working with the guiding precepts of right living. When we do business in a way in which everyone prospers and is nourished and rewarded, it is one of the highest ways of putting our spirituality to the test. The argument that a teacher asking for a fair exchange for services is not being spiritual is often a projection by the accuser, who is unwilling to be fair and equitable in his own dealings and is looking for justification for his own greed.

Generally Yoga teachers ask too little in exchange for their services, and this can be as ethically questionable as asking too much. Given our culture, asking too little can be a form of undervaluing the service and thus perpetuating a lack of value in the mind of the public. It is rare to see a Yoga class or workshop overpriced by regional standards. What may come into question, however, is not so much an equitable price for services but an equitable agreement as to when and how payment is made and if necessary when refunds should be offered.

Perhaps the matter would be clearer if we looked at how money is exchanged in other areas of our lives. How many of us would go to the grocery store, tell the checkout clerk that we forgot our wallet, and expect that we could take the groceries anyway? Can we enter a movie theater on the promise that we'll pay later? How many businesses would allow us to use their services for weeks at a time without prior payment? Yet this is often the situation Yoga teachers set up for themselves and contend with on an ongoing basis. When Yoga students are permitted to operate outside the parameters of what is fair within the culture, they are being taught to disrespect and undervalue the service they are receiving. Unfortunately lack of clarity about things financial can be a cause of real hardship for teachers. I believe that when we allow people to take something that is not freely offered, we are in essence encouraging the rudiments of stealing. A shoplifter who is not caught generally continues to shoplift. Similarly we do students no favor by allowing an unfair financial exchange to continue.

Many years ago a student attending public classes at the center where I worked made it a habit to come early and get, in effect, a thirty-minute private lesson for her physical problems. At the time I lacked clarity about my own boundaries and agreements and allowed this to continue, believing I was offering a valuable service. This student was wealthy and could certainly have afforded a private lesson, but she always had a reason for not doing so. It became clear through her interactions with other practitioners that she was accustomed to abusing the generosity of others, for instance by canceling massage appointments at a moment's notice (or with no notice at all) and in effect stealing that person's time and potential income. Allowing this behavior to continue was only unwittingly honing her skills in stealing from others. But more important, allowing myself to have my generosity abused was a way of undervaluing my service.

At other times, stealing can take a more subtle form. Susan, who lived in a luxurious home and made no secret of her fabulous lifestyle, always seemed to have a negative comment when it came time to pay for her classes. "I've done nothing but make out checks all day!" she would groan. Or "Oh God, it's payday again?" Her undermining comments left me feeling robbed of my dignity. This continued for many months until finally, after one particularly tactless comment, I asked her to put away her checkbook. When she seemed surprised I said, "I'm concerned that you're not getting what you need from these classes because your comments seem to imply they are not of value to you." When she expressed confusion, I continued, "I'm not sure whether you are aware of it, but every time you pay for your classes you make a comment that undermines my sense of dignity and worth. I would rather you stop paying for classes if you truly feel they are not worth the fee." This took her aback, and she adamantly expressed her appreciation for the classes. I was relieved that she never again made such comments.

One thing that has become clear to me in almost twenty-five years of teaching, and in listening to the financial dilemmas of my colleagues, is that establishing clear financial terms is only half the equation. If a teacher or director expresses these terms with even the smallest inkling of reticence, ambivalence, or apology, in that moment she is actively undermining the very agreements she has set forth. Even the subtlest unconscious discomfort about asking for fair remuneration will be interpreted by many students as a loophole through which they can circumvent a financial agreement. Peers who have shared stories of how students have accused them of "not being spiritual" when they have refused to extend a class card, or declined a refund, or simply asked for payment on time often feel perversely guilty of these accusations. Conversely I have noticed that colleagues who are clear about their financial terms and have no compunction about asking for payments rarely experience these kinds of interactions with their students. I believe this is because these teachers have prepared a ground in which these interactions cannot take root.

Generally studios that operate almost solely on a casual or drop-in basis leave themselves at the mercy of a fickle public and thereby leave their teachers in a very insecure financial situation. Those that do offer class cards to be used within a certain time frame can work if the time frame is enforced. Often however studios find themselves in regular negotiations with students who wish to extend their class cards beyond the expiration date for all manner of questionable reasons. Making sure that a student fully understands the terms of a class card arrangement prior to purchase and having those terms clearly printed on the card, along with an explicit statement that class cards cannot be extended, is one way of preventing students from trying to finagle exceptions.

A far more secure and equitable financial arrangement is to request prepayment and preregistration for Yoga courses (whether these be ongoing in four-to-eight-week periods or exclusive). In my own experience of running a center, I found that inevitably there were people who wanted to be on a registration list without paying and who would swear on the Bible that they would be there at the opening class. Many of these students would fail to turn up, often after we had turned away potential registrants. This meant that we lost much-needed income and that the people who had betrayed our trust had also in effect taken a place away from another student. This happened so often, for public classes, retreats, and teacher trainings, that the teachers at the center finally generated the policy that all registrants for a class must be paid in full to be truly registered for that class. When you ask people to make a financial commitment, you not only declare the value of the service you are offering but you also ask the students to recognize the value of what they are going to receive.

This policy works equally well for longer workshops and trainings, with the total amount due by an agreed-upon date, after which students are notified that they are at risk of being taken off the registration list. It is only fair to have a clearly stated cancellation and refund policy up front. This needs to be made explicit and in writing so there can be no misunderstanding later. Centers can consider a date before which cancellation is possible (with an administration fee deducted from the refund) and whether there will be no refund if the person's place cannot be filled from a waiting list after a certain date. Depending on the class or event, you must decide a reasonable time frame within which it is possible to take alternative registrants. Teachers who mostly teach private lessons need to decide their own policies. Some have a cancellation policy stated on their business card or brochure, such as "Please be aware that if you cancel your appointment with less than twenty-four hours' notice you will be charged 50 percent of your lesson fee" (or whatever seems fair). Often this is enough to make private students particularly respectful of the time they have booked. Having a cancellation policy can radically reduce the frequency of cancellations.

ETHICAL INQUIRY:
LATE PAYMENTS

This inquiry was contributed by a colleague.

"The day had finally come for me to advertise for my first Yoga class. The first difficulty I encountered was setting a price. As a new teacher, I felt that I couldn't ask a high price for the class, so I set the prices based on how much it would cost to rent the studio space and nothing more. The class filled quickly, with the majority of the students being close personal friends. I had more people wanting to take the Yoga class than I had space for, so I made a registration list and turned other students away. A week before the class started, I phoned everyone advising them of where to go and what to bring. Unfortunately many who had agreed to come now weren't so keen, and my numbers dwindled down so they barely covered the cost of the rent. I started to panic at the thought that I would have to pay to teach my first Yoga class! In the end, I had just enough people to cover the cost of the class.

"The next problem I encountered was getting the payment from all my friends/students. This part was tough. I felt embarrassed to ask my friends for money for my Yoga class, as this was my first teaching experience. Some of them paid straight away with no problem, but there were some that still hadn't paid halfway through the course, even though I continued to ask for payment. Since they were my friends, I felt it was important to remind them that their payment was to cover the cost of the studio space and was not for my own profit. It was a tough situation, as I didn't want to jeopardize any friendships, and I also didn't want to be stuck with the bill at the end of the day. I struggled with one particular student who I reminded about the payment every week. There were some weeks that he didn't show up at all. I felt incredibly guilty for having to ask for the full payment even though he didn't come to all the classes. I had to continually remind myself that if he signed up for the class and didn't come, it was his problem and not my own. That only made me feel a little bit better, but it was frustrating to know that a friend was not respecting my Yoga class or me. This has been a continuing problem, as the friend/student still hasn't paid for the class."

How might this teacher have prevented some of these problems from arising? How have her feelings about and discomfort with her own payment policy contributed to the ongoing challenge of nonpayment?

ETHICAL INQUIRY:
CHANGING THE TERMS
OF A MONETARY AGREEMENT

In the early years of teaching guest workshops, my class numbers were often very small, and sometimes the financial remuneration was low, especially when one factored in the time and energy of traveling to and from an engagement. Being paid modestly didn't concern me, as I realized I was getting invaluable experience, and I loved my work, whether well-paid or not. After two engagements at one Yoga center, the numbers began to increase until, for the third visit, we had a capacity attendance. I was thrilled, both for myself and for the director of the center.

As the workshop came to a close, the director invited a number of her regular students and me to dinner. To my astonishment, during the dinner and in front of the students, the director began questioning the terms of our written and signed contract. She asked whether there shouldn't be a ceiling on how much a visiting teacher earns and posed other questions to indicate that she felt I was taking more than was fair. I quickly told her that these were not issues I was willing to discuss at that time. Later, even though we had agreed to work on a percentage basis, she attempted to change the agreement and, when this didn't work, added expenses that had not been agreed upon, such as income lost through cancelled classes.

When it came time for me to leave, she handed me a check in such an ungracious manner that it was clear she felt cheated. I was pleased that I had not capitulated to her terms, which I knew to be unfair. I had not asked her for additional monies for the two previous engagements, which were poorly paid yet had taken just as much time and energy on my part, and now she was asking me for more money for a successful event in which she would duly share in the rewards. Her accusations of my greed were clearly a projection of her own greediness in taking more than her share. These maneuvers seemed all the more extraordinary because she had just returned from an expensive holiday in Europe, something I could only imagine in my dreams. I decided, upon reflection, never to teach at her center again because I did not believe we had a shared value about agreements.

While it was important in this instance not to budge from an agreement, there have been other instances when an organizer has come to me expressing that, because of increased numbers for a workshop, there has been an increase in time needed to administer the event. Because I have organized retreats through my office, I know just how complicated a large event can become. Although I was not legally bound to change the terms, in these instances I have gladly given a host more money to compensate for the additional work. This is another example of how the operation of an internal locus can help us to determine a right action in the context of a given situation. ◼ ◼

ETHICAL INQUIRY:
OPERATING A VIABLE BUSINESS
WHILE OFFERING TEACHINGS OF INTEGRITY

This inquiry was contributed by a colleague.

"Never compromise compassion, kindness, and care for money. For example, we run five-dollar classes three times every weekday. We make no profit from these classes whatsoever, but here's why they work:

- The Yoga teachers are still paid a normal, fair rate for teaching the class.
- Yoga becomes available to members of the community who couldn't otherwise afford it.
- We have an unbelievably strong reputation in the community as a result of these classes, and people travel significant distances to come to them.
- Many students who attend these classes have gone on to attend retreats, other higher-cost classes, and even to complete teacher training (so it works a bit like a loss leader in a supermarket).
- The studio has lots of people coming through every day, all of whom add vibrant energy and contribute to our *satsang*.

"My practice on the mat and running a business is an ever-evolving, ever-deepening opportunity to get closer to truly understanding that we are all one and there truly is no separation between us. Whatever you bring to your practice on the mat gets amplified. If you bring ego and selfish ambition to your practice, that is what tends to grow. If you bring an intention of peace for all beings, that will gradually expand and begin to fill your life and the lives of those around you. It's the same with running a business. Intention is everything. You will make mistakes, and there will be casualties along the way, but with an intention of upliftment and kindness you can't go far wrong. If you go into the Yoga field looking to become rich quick, you're in the wrong place. After years of working in this industry, I don't know anyone who is rolling in money. In fact most of studio owners and teachers I know still wonder how they will pay the rent next month, and it's often the same for us. But I do know many fulfilled and gracious individuals who couldn't imagine doing anything else. It is a true blessing to make your living doing something you love, and each time I open the doors in the morning or get up to teach a class, I try to remember that every student who comes to the studio is a holy being and it is an honor that they are there."

This teacher is an inspiring friend, teacher, and business owner. In my conversations with her, she has expressed her belief that the bottom line in running a Yoga business should be offering teachings of integrity. Her experience is that when we make the teachings our foremost concern, the prosperity of the business will follow. Notice what factors enter into your own decision-making process when running your Yoga business. Are there ways you can make the teachings of Yoga more widely available to your community?

REFUNDS

It is only fair that if a person cancels at such a late date that another cannot fill his place, he loses his money. That said, when a student has had to cancel because of an act of God, such as an illness, an accident, or a death, it can be just as important to show good will in giving him a refund. When considering a student's request for a refund, it is important to look at the specific context and situation to decide what is fair to both parties.

ETHICAL INQUIRY: REFUND POLICIES

Just prior to a recent teacher training, a registrant discovered that her mother was very ill. Because she could not have controlled or foreseen this situation, we offered her a refund, and she was so grateful that she asked to have the money applied to the following year's training. We took her expressed attitude into consideration: she said that she knew about the cancellation policy, she understood and respected it, and she and would be happy with whatever we decided.

At the same time, an individual showed up for the introductory evening and at the end, having not attended one class, decided to cancel. We had a long waiting list, but at such late notice no one could be expected to reorganize her life to attend a long training. Additionally the person was quite aggressive and demanding about receiving a refund. We offered him the opportunity to stay for three days and then, should he still feel the same way, we would refund for the remainder of the training. But this offer was rejected and, given that he had not been willing to give us a chance, we felt no compelling reason to go against our clearly stated cancellation policy. We reasoned that it was his responsibility to adequately research the investment he made in the training, and there was nothing in his application that gave us cause for concern. We made it a point to review all applications carefully for the very purpose of screening out registrants who might find the training unsuitable to their goals, and we erred on the side of caution and declined some applicants. With all these factors in mind, in this instance we decided to adhere to our cancellation policy.

As you can see, deciding what is ethical involves not only having a clearly stated agreement but also taking each case and its context into consideration. While we were not legally obliged to provide a refund to either participant, we arrived at two very different conclusions, both of which we felt were ethically correct. ■ ■

WORK–STUDY AND SCHOLARSHIPS

Most Yoga studios and teachers strongly believe in and implement plans to allow those with financial hardship to study. It can be immensely satisfying to see an individual who might otherwise not have had a chance to receive teachings benefit from financial assistance. In speaking with directors of other centers, it's clear that coming up with a fair policy on this matter is fraught with difficulty, because it is not always simple to discern who is truly in need of help. In my early years of offering unassessed scholarships to students, I was frequently chagrined by people who pleaded poverty to get a scholarship and then made massage and manicure appointments for themselves during a training and headed for restaurants every evening. On one occasion I was informed that a scholarship student had to leave a training early to get to her Italian skiing holiday on time! After being burned one too many times, it became clear that not carefully assessing scholarship requests not only made for an unfair exchange for the teacher but also prevented the center from being able to help truly needy students.

Because of the context of the culture in which we live and the general belief that anything of worth costs money, it can often be simpler to offer someone a work exchange for a course. In this way there is some kind of energetic exchange. It is important for all people's dignity and self-respect to be able to reciprocate in some form. In setting up a work exchange agreement, however, the job description, time frame for work done, and other terms of exchange need to be explicit and agreed upon prior to the work commencing. It is also important to verify that the person earnestly wants to study Yoga and is going to take the work exchange just as seriously. There is nothing more annoying than spending weeks training someone to do a job and then having her decide that Yoga is really not her thing after all. Sometimes the very causes of someone's inability to pay for a course are indicative of a confused and chaotic life, so work–study exchanges should be entered into with a wary eye. On the other end of the spectrum, when someone has been too ill to work in exchange for a course, I often look for some small task (such as setting up the altar each day or tidying a tea and refreshment table) that will enable him to feel he is contributing something.

The matter of scholarships is somewhat more complicated. At the very least an application and screening process where fair assessment can be made needs to be put in place. Another way of addressing scholarship potential is assessment based as much on merit as on need. This system has worked well at many centers, where a student who has already proven her seriousness, her work ethic, and her integrity is given a scholarship to allow her to study further or in more depth than she would be able to do under her own steam. Generally these are students who would walk over broken glass to study Yoga, and they are often people who would turn themselves inside out to pay for a course. Often recipients of scholarships are single mothers and fathers, or people fraught with medical bills for their children or relatives, or simply those from poor circumstances who have had few opportunities to improve themselves. My own professional policy now with scholarships is that I (or my host for a workshop or intensive) must already know the student and must have prior knowledge of the student's sincerity. I believe that this is very important, because when we wantonly throw our generosity away to the wrong people, we also inadvertently deny deserving people.

Being ethical always involves looking at the larger context of a situation. In our culture people often believe it is a right rather than a luxury to eat out at restaurants, buy expensive clothing, go on holidays, have every object they desire, and still be able to do whatever they want to do. The idea of making a sacrifice in order to embark on a period of study is becoming a rather rare notion. In these instances the student would like the center or teacher to make the sacrifice, which is clearly an unbalanced arrangement. In the years of my own training, I lived with others in a rented house, had few items of clothing, rarely ate out, and either rode my bike to class or took public transportation (often late at night). Curiously I did not feel poor because I was pouring my heart and mind into something I loved and believed in. It never occurred to me to request a scholarship, because I had always worked for my education. But I did any number of work exchange jobs to pay my fees, from licking stamps and sealing envelopes to typing letters and putting away chairs. My background has obviously shaped my attitude and stance about work exchange and scholarships, but it has not prevented me from assessing the merits of each case in as objective a way as I can.

There are instances however when the only right thing to do is to offer one's teaching without any financial compensation. I have given master classes for teachers for free when the attendees all offered their own teaching voluntarily as community service. I have worked privately with very sick and in some cases terminally ill students for no fee. It is not only honorable to do so, it is a privilege to work with someone throughout an illness and prior to death. The enormous learning experience this can offer is worth its weight in gold. Selfless service can be the ultimate satisfaction, and no other exchange is necessary in these instances.

Sutra II.40

When cleanliness is developed it reveals what needs to be constantly maintained and what is eternally clean. What decays is external. What does not is deep within us.

Appropriate Dress for the Teacher

When we enter a Yoga studio, ashram, or center as teachers, our role is to be of service to the student and also to create a safe and sacred environment for study. By dressing modestly and in a way that does not distract, we help the students focus on their own inner perceptions and the content of what is being taught. When teaching asana, it is important that the students be able to clearly see the teacher's body, but this can be achieved without unnecessarily sexualizing the body. Wearing clothing that reveals too much cleavage or is cut so low as to reveal the label on one's underwear can be distracting if not embarrassing to some students. Wearing shorts that allow the genitals to be inadvertently exposed (especially for male teachers) or fabric that is so sheer as to be see-though are other things to be aware of. Selecting clothing with political slogans or wild patterns or colors can also draw attention away from the study at hand and toward the teacher and his fashion sense.

One particular teacher comes to mind. She dressed for class in what can only be described as an imitation of a French prostitute, with velvet neck chokers, glittering, dangling earrings, and wrists layered with bangles. She would adorn herself with garish and multicolored fabrics, often lacy, and revealing, low-cut tops. On one occasion her sheer pantyhose left an entire group of students slack-jawed when she demonstrated Half Downward-Facing Dog Pose (Ardha Adho Mukha Svanasana) and revealed more than anyone wished to see. When confronted by the director of the center, she gushed, "But this is who I am! This is my self-expression." Clearly when self-expression is considered more important than the students' needs, the teacher's values need to be reprioritized. In this instance the director decided to put in place a clear dress code.

Teachers also need to reflect on whether their choice of dress in any way, whether consciously or unconsciously, communicates a desire for and availability as an intimate partner. Our appearance communicates to the world at large our personal boundaries and is an invitation to either respect those boundaries or transgress them. In the previous example, the Yoga teacher's dress sense indicated larger boundary issues. At the conclusion of a seminar hosted for an Indian teacher of extremely high reputation, the crowd stood aghast when she came up behind the teacher and wrapped her arms around him, kissing him on the neck as a goodbye gesture. For any teacher, but especially a married teacher from a very traditional background, this uninvited public display of affection was deeply perturbing. In the end the director felt she could no longer have this teacher teaching at her center.

Certainly when we enter an ashram or community where there is a clear dress code, we should adhere to that code out of respect for the place we are entering. Often this involves wearing loose-fitting cotton clothing that specifically does not reveal the body.

When considering what to wear to and from class and during class, ask yourself whether, as a teacher, what you are wearing serves to clarify your teaching or detract from it. When teaching a spinal-care class, a teacher may choose to wear a leotard that allows the back muscles to be clearly revealed. The same teacher might wear a long-sleeved shirt and loose-fitting pants when teaching a meditation class. We should be clear that our decision to dress modestly has nothing to do with prudery or outdated Victorian morality and everything to do with our primary imperative as a teacher. It is possible to dress elegantly and attractively, in a way that makes class a pleasant experience for everyone. The class should never be about the teacher or his trappings but about the content of what the teacher has to offer.

ETHICAL INQUIRY: DRESSED IN A THONG

A few years ago I sprained my ankle badly prior to a teaching tour. While attending a large Yoga conference, I decided to sit in on a number of classes to observe and learn from the other presenters. Sitting in the corner of the room where the class was about to begin, I noticed that it was five minutes past the starting time. The male teacher then entered and strutted confidently down the center of the room to the front, where he dropped his sweat pants and stood before a crowd of more than fifty people revealing naked buttocks in a pair of thong underwear. Strangely he then put his yoga shorts over the top of his thong and proceeded to teach class. None of the students commented, which did not surprise me, given the authoritative way in which he had dropped his drawers, as if this were a perfectly normal way to begin teaching. After class I noticed that the men's bathroom was adjacent to the conference room, so it would have been easy to change there. A number of my colleagues who were in attendance came up to share their disgust at the inappropriate nature of the teacher's opening gesture. I felt compelled to share my concerns with the conference director, who to my great surprise did not take exception to this behavior until I communicated that a number of the participants had stated their shock to me after the class. I am certain that, had a female teacher given a similar display, she would have been confronted within the day, and news of her behavior would have quickly traveled within the Yoga community.

Consider whether you would think it strange, or find it uncomfortable, for your high school physical education teacher, your doctor, or your lawyer, to strip down to his underwear and change his clothes in front of you. Would you be uncomfortable with your Yoga teacher doing this? If not, why not? If so, explain your reasoning. Do you think there are gender inequities within the Yoga community, and if so, how do they manifest? ▨ ▨

Appropriate Dress for the Student

While it is important in an asana class to be able to see a student's body, not all students feel comfortable dressing in close-fitting clothing. This can be especially true for overweight students, who may feel embarrassed enough just coming to class. Additionally some people's religious or cultural beliefs may place restrictions on how they dress (for instance, Mormons and Muslims). On the other end of the spectrum, more and more young students attend class in clothing that would be more suited to the nightclub or the singles scene at a local bar. It is always easier to make a request known to a group than it is to single out an individual. As one of my dear Sufi friends used to say, "Sometimes it's best to wrap one's bitter message in humor." We might ask that women refrain from wearing yoga pants that expose thongs or G-strings out of respect for others, who have not agreed to view the student's personal lingerie collection.

We should also be respectful in asking a student to take off an outer layer of clothing to demonstrate a movement more clearly for the group. And we should always ask permission to adjust a student's clothing (for instance, when we need to see a segment of the spinal column). A teacher once pulled my pants down below the crack of my buttocks in front of an entire group and launched into a description of my lumbar spine, without it occurring to him that it was inappropriate to adjust my clothing or touch an intimate part of my body without my permission.

A more frequently voiced concern is the issue of cleanliness and in particular strong body odor. In many instances students have told me after class that another student's body odor was unbearable but they were too embarrassed to tell the other person. I have heard similar stories from flummoxed colleagues. It can be particularly awkward to address this issue one-to-one, so my suggestion is to make a tactful announcement at the beginning of the course, especially if you are entering a hot time of the year, when body odor and perspiration become more of an issue. One can also put friendly suggestions in the changing rooms and bathrooms to "Freshen up prior to class to make class a pleasant experience for everyone." Then support the notice by leaving unscented baby wipes, paper towels, and unscented deodorants for communal use. When this strategy doesn't send the message to a particular individual, it really is best to gently broach the subject privately. Be mindful that she may have a health issue that is causing her bad breath or body odor, such as a liver problem or other infection, and this may be important information for the teacher to know. While handling such issues is not always easy, whenever a student is having a negative effect upon the group's ability to learn, it is the teacher's responsibility to rectify the situation.

FOUL LANGUAGE

Teachers need to be mindful that language they use in private may offend when used in the context of a Yoga class. In keeping with this, while humor can lighten a class, dirty jokes are generally are not a good idea. Students also need to be aware that a Yoga studio or ashram is a sacred space for spiritual practice, and language that may be perfectly fine to use outside the Yoga studio in casual conversation is often not appropriate inside the practice room.

A colleague recently related a story about a renowned teacher visiting her city. On the Friday evening that was to begin the weekend intensive, the room was packed with students sitting quietly in meditation. When the teacher entered the room, he started by saying: "You lot are fucking keen! In America they'd be lying down by now." The students were flabbergasted at this offensive greeting, and they were equally disturbed that his instruction for the next ninety minutes was peppered with similarly foul language. As my colleague said, "Of course, I occasionally use such language myself, as I'm sure everyone in the room does, but when you are doing your spiritual practice it is particularly off-putting to hear someone continually swearing." The next day attendance dropped to eight people. Students had voted with their feet and clearly would not tolerate being spoken to in this manner, regardless of how famous the teacher was.

SUTRA II.36

When one abides in truthfulness, activity and its fruition
are grounded in the truth.

CONFIDENTIALITY

The word *confidential* implies that we have another's trust or confidence to uphold. When a student comes to study with us, we need to be aware that what transpires within the classroom or private class setting is to be held in trust. Talking about a student to another student, using a student's name in casual public conversation, or publicly divulging information about a student's health, progress, or personal issues undermines the trust that has been vested in us. Some of the ethics to consider here include:

- Refraining from referring to the student by his or her name in a public or private forum.

- Asking the student's permission to speak about her concerns or condition with a member of her family, another teacher, or a health professional.
- Refraining from speaking about the student to another person in a tone, manner, or with words that we would not use to the student directly. This practice in particular can cultivate an abiding respect for the student's process.

Often when teachers speak about a student to others, it is because they lack awareness of the potential harm that such casual conversation can do. When you feel at risk of breaching confidentiality, you might pause and ask yourself if you would still feel okay about what you are saying if the student were to discover the nature and content of your conversation. Just as often, the teacher may lack a peer group or mentor with whom to discuss difficult issues and questions that are arising in relationship to a particular student. Instead of discussing the student within the bounds of a professional relationship, the teacher may begin to have leaky boundaries and allow such discussion to overflow into his personal life.

During my teacher-training programs, my coteacher, my assistants, and I meet regularly at lunch and in the evenings throughout the training. If a particular student is of concern, we discuss that student within the privacy of the meeting. We then mentally circle that individual as a special-attention person, and someone is designated to check in with the person each day to discern, as best they can, how the person is progressing. Neither the student nor any other member of the group is aware that they have been designated as a special-attention case. If they have shared personal information with a particular assistant and the assistant feels the information would be useful to the teacher's group, then the assistant asks permission to share that information with the other teachers. Similarly if a student has shared an intimate detail of his physical history with me, I ask permission to bring the case to the group's attention so we might learn together.

For instance, if a student has just told me about her spinal problem and I believe my work with her would be useful for the rest of the group to view, I might first ask "Would you be comfortable with me sharing details about your spinal problem with the group? Would you be comfortable demonstrating in front of the group?" Although it does not happen often, there have been instances when students have expressed to me that they do not want details of their physical problems aired in front of others, and in these instances it is important to respect that individual's wishes.

The need for and practice of confidentiality comes as second nature to those working within professions where it is not only unethical to breach confidentiality but also illegal. The psychiatrist or psychotherapist is practiced at upholding strict confidentiality about her clients. The doctor working in a health clinic cannot tell a friend about a mutual friend's visit to the clinic, let alone speak about the nature of what transpired. The priest does not divulge what is said in the confessional. Yoga teachers, while not legally bound to uphold confidentiality, often wear multiple professional hats that are similar in capacity to other service professions. Recently a colleague (who is also an acupuncturist) notified me that one of the students in my teacher training was having difficulty and that it may be related to her past. She did not state whether the woman had been her patient but said that I might want to investigate further. When questioned she could only say that the "student herself will have to tell you." Many months later the student did indeed discuss her struggle with drug addiction, and it was clear that this information could only be divulged by her and at a time when she was ready to share it. I appreciated the way my colleague respected her confidentiality agreement. It would have been easy to provide details, especially because the student involved was quite a popular teacher within the community, and the information might have been considered prime gossip material. Her integrity in holding the information modeled a standard to which many of us as Yoga teachers might aspire.

When you feel at risk of breaching a student's confidentiality, you might pause and reflect whether your words or actions might be regretted later.

Would you still feel okay about your behavior if the person involved found out? You can also ask yourself how you would feel if a teacher spoke about you without permission.

SUTRA 1.8

Incorrect knowledge is a false understanding not
based on the true nature of what is perceived.

SPEAKING ABOUT OTHER TEACHERS OR METHODS

Teachers are often put in the position of being asked about another teacher, another Yoga method, and even a divergent technical point about how an asana should be practiced. The simplest way to determine a course of action here is to follow the old adage of treating others as you wish to be treated yourself. Consider how you would feel if you discovered that another teacher spoke disparagingly about your work in front of a group of students, cast aspersions on a technique you practice outside the context in which it was used, or damned your method of Yoga without having had direct experience of that method. When students ask me what I think about another teacher or a technique that another teacher recommends, I generally respond that I cannot comment on what another teacher has done or understand the reasoning behind her technique outside the context of its use. What I can share with them is my own reasoning for using a particular technique and my own peda-gogic model for teaching. I then ask the student to be the judge of what is most useful and relevant to him. I make it a practice never to speak badly about another teacher in front of a group of students.

When a student has asked about another Yoga method, I generally recommend that the best way to find out about a method is to experience it firsthand, that is, for the student to make her own investigation. If I have knowledge of a method, I may describe some of the key features, stating that every method has its strengths and weaknesses and also that a method is only as good as the teacher who teaches it. I would not hesitate however to privately caution an individual student if I believed that a particular method might be unsuitable for him at that time. For instance a student with high blood pressure might be cautioned to avoid a method in which the room was heated to an elevated temperature and the practices were vigorous.

When I have firsthand knowledge that a teacher has an unresolved history of unethical behavior or I have strong reason to believe a teacher is working in an unsound or injurious fashion, this can put me in an ethical quandary. Not to warn a student is to risk putting her in harm's way. Usually such questions are asked in private, and generally I say, "I can't recommend that teacher." A student who has worked with me for some time will generally accept that answer, realizing that I would not make such a statement without due cause. If a student presses for further information, I might be compelled to share that I have direct knowledge of "unresolved unethical behavior." While I might have direct knowledge of many students being injured by a teacher or of sexual indiscretions by a teacher, it is rarely necessary to say more than "I have concerns." It is then up to the student to do her own investigation and come to her own conclusions.

ETHICAL INQUIRY: NAME-DROPPING

Louise decided to attend an introductory meditation class for one evening. The visiting teacher, who was billed as a famous expert from afar, sprinkled his discourse with comments about his past students, name-dropping all the celebrities who had worked privately with him. After telling the class how one celebrity had a habit of falling asleep in meditation class, and how another had great trouble with certain practices, Louise was not so sure she wanted to work with this teacher. She wondered whether her name might come up in casual conversation at some other center, or whether the intimate details of her meditation practice might be divulged elsewhere. She also wondered whether the teacher was shamelessly promoting himself to the detriment of the teaching and whether his frequent mentions of the "need for private lessons" was a ploy to make more money. Based on this one experience, she decided not to work further with this teacher. ■ ■

ETHICAL INQUIRY:
A TEACHER SPEAKS TO HIS
STUDENTS ABOUT ANOTHER STUDENT

While attending a month-long Yoga intensive, Barbara discovered that the teacher had been talking about her to a number of other students, in particular making disparaging comments about her practice. Because the teacher had not first come to her with these concerns, she felt particularly violated. Unbeknownst to the teacher, Barbara had been struggling with frightening dreams during the intensive as well as with health problems that would not have been obvious to anyone else. When she found out the teacher had so casually commented on her "emotional blocks," she felt unable to continue as a member of the group. By speaking about her without her permission, the teacher had separated her from the group, making the other students confidants and her the outsider. When she asked to speak with the teacher about the matter privately after class, the teacher said she was the only person who had learned nothing in almost three weeks, and that if she weren't so emotionally blocked she would be able to do the advanced backbends. Having had her internal process so brutally judged left her devastated, and on reflection she decided to leave the retreat. ■ ■

SUTRA II.31

These universal moral principles [yamas], unrestricted by conditions
of birth, place, time or circumstance, are the great vow of yoga.'

ETHICAL CODES

It could be said that the Yoga tradition has as clear a code of ethics as any situation would require. Patanjali does indeed outline ten clear precepts for
rightful living in his yamas and niyamas presented in the Yoga Sutra. But the
information is skeletal and therefore is prone to a high degree of variation in
interpretation. This perhaps reflects the internal locus principle that asks us to
consider, moment to moment, within the context of a particular situation,
whether an action is ethical or unethical. Most professions provide their
members with a clear external locus as well, in the form of a code of ethics.
Having a clear code serves to give a group, organization, business, or community a shared set of values to uphold and clear parameters for determining
when a member is not adhering to those values.

At the time of this writing, there is no agreed-upon national or international
code of ethics governing the Yoga profession. Because there is no formal code,
transgressions, even extreme transgressions, are unable to be processed intelligently. Because there is no umbrella organization that acts as a registry, there
is also no clearinghouse for complaints to be aired. What is ethical is therefore
left completely up to individual interpretation, something that would not be
acceptable in the fields of education, medicine, or other professions similar to
our own.

We can however, as individuals within our community, make a grassroots
effort to establish a clear code of ethics. Directors of Yoga centers can establish their own codes, make these codes known and understood by the staff,
and create a protocol for handling complaints. Directors of ashrams and
retreat venues can insist upon teachers' adherence to the code as a prerequi-

site to their being able to work at that center. Similarly conference organizers can make a code of ethics part of the contractual agreement that guest teachers sign prior to teaching at a Yoga conference. There are now some Yoga centers that make a code of conduct part of the contract signed by visiting teachers and have boards to handle ethical queries. This is a clear way of creating and sustaining the integrity of a sacred place in which people can do transformational work.

Teachers too, especially those of us who train teachers or who have the privilege of traveling to share knowledge with other centers, can use our power to insist that any center that we visit not only have a code of ethics but adhere to that code. Several years ago I decided to turn my feelings of despair into strength through action. Disheartened about the abysmal state of affairs that was causing our community's dirty laundry to be aired on the front pages of national newspapers, I decided to inform all my hosts at centers worldwide that I would no longer teach at any center that knowingly continued to host a teacher with established and unresolved unethical behavior. This did three things. First it sent a clear message that my teaching at their center was contingent upon certain values. Next it sent a clear message to those who had been harmed by unethical behavior that "business as usual" was not an acceptable response to unethical behavior. And finally it simplified and improved my own teaching relationships, because I weeded out those centers with which I did not have shared values. Despite warnings from colleagues that this would have dire financial consequences for me, placing this condition on my hosts did not affect me adversely, either personally or professionally. To the contrary, many centers that had benefited financially from my workshops and master classes were the financial losers.

It is unfortunate but true that financial consequences, whether in the form of a boycott or through political leveraging, is one of the most powerful tools for social change and one of the most important deterrents to unethical behavior. When a doctor or lawyer considers the consequences of losing her ability to make her livelihood from a profession that has taken years of invest-ment to establish, this is undoubtedly a strong deterrent to casual or wanton disregard of ethical conduct. Within the Yoga profession there have been few consequences to unethical behavior. When teachers continue to receive guest teaching engagements and invitations to deliver keynote addresses at major Yoga conferences regardless of their unethical behavior, this sends a resound-ing message throughout the community. In denying, ignoring, covering up, or rationalizing such behavior (some of which would be considered illegal and cause for deregistration in other professions), we act in complicity with the perpetrators and actively encourage them to continue to act unethically. We should be aware as a community that to turn a blind eye when there is some-thing that we can do to prevent further harm is to incur our own karmic debt. Many women have corresponded with me throughout the years, telling me their stories about unethical behavior. They have communicated that the denial, ostracism, and lack of action on the part of the Yoga community in response to their claims has done as much if not more harm to them than the actions of the perpetrator.

Senior teachers, especially those who have the power to draw large num-bers of students, have considerable clout, which they can use to change the sit-uation. I have often thought that if only ten major touring teachers placed this condition upon their hosting centers, we would see a vast reduction in the number of unethical teachers who continue not only to be supported but to be rewarded for their damaging behavior. It is a political power however that has yet to be utilized.

What follows is an excellent and well-considered code of ethics, gener-ated by the Yoga Research and Education Center (YREC). I encourage you to look closely at each point and, if you are a director, to consider having a meeting with your teachers to go over the code and consider adopting it for your center.

Ethical Guidelines for Yoga Teachers from the Yoga Research and Education Center

Yoga is an integrated way of life, which includes moral standards—traditionally called "virtues"—that any reasonable human being will find in principle acceptable. Some of these standards are encoded in the first limb *(anga)* of Patanjali's eightfold path (Ashtanga-yoga), called yama ("discipline" or "restraint"). According to Patanjali's *Yoga-Sutra*, this practice category is composed of the following five virtues:

- nonharming (ahimsa)
- truthfulness (satya)
- nonstealing (asteya)
- chastity (brahmacharya)
- greedlessness (aparigraha)

These have been explained by traditional authorities and also by modern interpreters.

In other key scriptures of Yoga, further moral principles are mentioned, including kindness, compassion, generosity, patience, helpfulness, forgiveness, purity, and so on. All these are virtues that we connect with a "good" person and which are demonstrated to a superlative degree in the lives of the great masters of Yoga.

In light of this, it seems appropriate for contemporary Yoga teachers to endeavor to conduct their lives in consonance with the moral principles put forward in Yoga. As teachers, they have a great responsibility toward their students, and they can be expected to clearly demonstrate the qualities one would associate with a good teacher. As practitioners and representatives of Yoga, their behavior can be expected to reflect the high moral standards espoused in Yoga. At the same time, we must take into account the present-day sociocultural context, which differs in some ways from the conditions of premodern India.

YREC views the formulation and publication of these ethical guidelines as part of its effort to help preserve the traditional legacy of Yoga and improve the quality of Yoga teaching and practice in the modern world.

1. Yoga teachers understand and appreciate that teaching Yoga is a noble and ennobling endeavor, which aligns them with a long line of honorable teachers.

2. Yoga teachers are committed to practicing Yoga as a way of life.

3. Yoga teachers are committed to maintaining impeccable standards of professional competence and integrity.

4. Yoga teachers dedicate themselves to a thorough and continuing study and practice of Yoga, in particular the theoretical and practical aspects of the branch or type of Yoga that they teach others.

5. Yoga teachers are committed to avoiding substance abuse and, if for some reason, they succumb to chemical dependency, will stop teaching until they are free again from drug and alcohol abuse. In that case, they will do everything in their power to stay free, including full accountability to a support group.

6. Yoga teachers will accurately represent their education, training, and experience relevant to their teaching of Yoga.

7. Yoga teachers are committed to promoting the physical, mental, and spiritual well-being of their students.

8. Yoga teachers, especially those teaching Hatha-Yoga, will abstain from giving medical advice, or advice that could be interpreted as such, unless they have the necessary medical qualifications.

9. Yoga teachers particularly embrace the ideal of truthfulness in dealing with students and others.

10. Yoga teachers are open to instructing all students irrespective of race, nationality, gender, sexual orientation, and social or financial status.

11. Yoga teachers are willing to accept students with physical disabilities, providing they have the skill to teach those students properly.

12. Yoga teachers will treat their students with respect.

13. Yoga teachers will never force their own opinions on students but appreciate the fact that every individual is entitled to his or her worldview, ideas, and beliefs. At the same time, however, Yoga teachers must communicate to their students that Yoga seeks to achieve a deep level of transformation of the human personality, including attitudes and ideas. If a student is not open to change, or if a student's opinions seriously impede the process of communicating yogic teachings to him or her, then the Yoga teacher is free to refuse to work with that individual and, if possible, find an amicable way of dissolving the teaching relationship.

14. Yoga teachers will avoid any form of sexual harassment of students.

15. Yoga teachers wishing to enter a consensual sexual relationship with a present or former student should seek the immediate counsel of their peers before taking any action.

16. Yoga teachers will make every effort to avoid exploiting the trust and potential dependency of students and instead encourage them to find greater inner freedom.

17. Yoga teachers acknowledge the importance of the proper context for teaching and agree to avoid teaching in a casual manner, which includes observing proper decorum inside and outside the class.

18. Yoga teachers strive to practice tolerance toward other Yoga teachers, schools, and traditions. When criticism has to be brought, this should be done in fairness and with appropriate regard for the facts.

These ethical guidelines are not exhaustive, and the fact that a given conduct is not specifically covered by these guidelines does not say anything about the ethical or unethical nature of that conduct. Yoga teachers always endeavor to respect and, to the best of their abilities, adhere to the traditional yogic code of conduct as well as to the law current in their country or state.[4]

Protocols for Handling Complaints

In other professions, one of the first actions taken when a person's behavior comes under question is to communicate this concern from peer to peer. This is the least threatening and confrontational option to an individual, giving her the opportunity to clarify her actions. It prevents what might have been a minor or "one-off" transgression from becoming a pattern. It also protects the reputation and integrity of the profession by not allowing a behavior to continue unchecked for so long that the first time peers hear of it is on the front page of a newspaper.

When peer-to-peer communication does not produce a satisfactory outcome, a Yoga center that has a clearly stated code of ethics (a prerequisite) has a number of options. If there is a board of advisors (ideally chosen from the most senior teachers within the community and not necessarily only from the center itself), the person may be asked to come before the board and explain his actions. It makes good sense for a Yoga center to form a board that includes members outside its own staff to reduce the possibility of a conflict of interest and increase the likelihood of objective decision-making. Such a board may have many options at its disposal, including:

Peer to peer confrontation. Although this is the most discreet first move, its disadvantage is that it may be difficult to discern whether the behavior is continuing in the future.

Formal reprimand and subsequent supervision. Continued employment can be made contingent upon no further reports of the stated behavior. The nature of the transgression would likely remain confidential, known only to the board and those effected.

Recommendation of counseling. In the case of drug, alcohol, or sexual addiction, the teacher may be advised to stop teaching until she has her addiction under control and has obtained support from a suitably qualified person. A member of the board or staff who has no conflict of interest may also be asked to act as a supervisor who meets with the person regularly to discuss her progress. Reinstatement of the teacher can be contingent on her taking full possession of herself and full responsibility to prevent further transgressions.

Removal. If a teacher shows no remorse for her behavior or is not able to give assurance that the behavior will stop, then the center has the option to remove that person from staff. Once a director or board has foreknowledge of unethical behavior, they may be held liable should a member of the public be harmed later. That is, if an illegal behavior (such as sexual molestation) has been clearly established and if a board has knowledge and denies or ignores such behavior, they may be liable should a member of the public subsequently lay charges. (Boards should check with the state and federal laws governing both profit and nonprofit boards.)

Censorship and Public Disclosure: A teacher may be severely reprimanded for her behavior and if necessary a full disclosure made to the local community or general public. In the case of one center that discovered their spiritual director had a long-standing history of sexual indiscretions, he was formally removed from office and a public statement was made about the nature of the abuse and the steps put in place to rectify any harm done.

Deregistration: In the case of a Yoga organization that does have a registry of members, a teacher may be deregistered and prevented in future from advertising himself as a member of the registry or organization.

Legal Action: When a behavior would be regarded as illegal in the eyes of the laws of a state or country, the most intelligent action for the board or director may be to make a formal police complaint. This is obviously an extreme action and not to be taken lightly or without legal counsel. However, it is far better than if a member of the public lays a complaint against the center itself.

ETHICAL INQUIRY:
VISITING TEACHERS

Roberta had run her own center for many years but was reluctant to put a code of ethics in place. She was unclear about whether to continue hosting teachers who had known histories of unresolved unethical behavior. These teachers were very popular and brought in significant revenue for her. She invited a guest teacher with whom she had no prior experience but who was reputedly "making waves" as a popular teacher.

Roberta became concerned on the first day of the workshop, because the teacher was clearly making overtures to the young female students, and she called him into her office to discuss the matter. Laughing, he declared that she was merely jealous that he was not showing her the same interest. It was clear to her at that moment that this man had no sense of the inappropriate nature of his behavior nor any desire to change the behavior, even at her request. Still not clear about a course of action, she decided to see the weekend out. After all, she reasoned, what harm could come from a short weekend workshop and private lessons?

By the end of the weekend, however, Roberta was informed by the local police that two women who had had private lessons with the guest teacher had filed complaints that they had been indecently assaulted. The police informed Roberta that, should the teacher still be within the city limits, he would be arrested.

At what point could Roberta have prevented this chain of events? Some possibilities are:

- Requiring that she or a member of her staff have prior experience with teachers before inviting them.
- Reviewing her criteria for hiring guest teachers and discerning between celebrities and reputable teachers with valuable information to share with her students.
- Requiring that visiting teachers sign a contract that includes a code of ethics.

- Terminating the contract with the teacher as soon as she saw his unethical behavior.

Roberta is now working on a code of ethics for her staff. She is aware that she has a responsibility to her students to bring only reputable teachers to her center and a responsibility to ensure their physical, emotional, and psychological safety. ◼ ◼

OPENING DOORS

Throughout the writing of this book, I have been struck by the complex nature of ethical inquiry. It seems that each question opens a door to another question, which often requires deeper inspection and reveals yet another layer of understanding. The generous contributions of stories and questions from students, colleagues, and peers opened my eyes to issues that I had not considered and at times opened my attitude to an issue that might have previously provoked a dogmatic reaction in me. It is my hope that this small book prompts introspection and discussion of ethical issues within the worldwide Yoga community.

The issues raised in this book are by no means exhaustive. If a given ethical concern is not specifically addressed here, I hope that the principles discussed will help with its resolution. The principles outlined here are meant to help you, as teacher or student, to navigate your way through new and challenging situations.

The transplantation of the Yoga tradition from an Eastern to a Western culture can only be successful if we integrate the highest ethical teachings of the tradition into the context of our own societal mores. While it is true that the consumerism, commercialization, and a breakdown of values in our culture are strong forces that run contrary to this integration, our culture does hold values that support ethical clarity and ethical action. For instance, our culture has a collective clarity about the fair exchange of money, and we can use that clarity in our spiritual practice. Our culture has clear laws in place to prevent and deter sexual harassment within our institutions. We also have clear laws governing matters of confidentiality and professional propriety that we can use as guidelines for our own profession. Let us not muddy this clarity by rationalizing, covering up, or ignoring unethical behavior because it has taken place in a spiritual context. Rather, it is the spiritual context itself that requires of us an even greater commitment to live ethically. It is this uncompromising reverence for life, manifested through our thoughts, speech and actions, that can lead not only to our own peace and freedom but to a world that is peaceful and free.

PART III

TEACHER'S WORKBOOK: RESOLVING ETHICAL ISSUES

A Working Model

WHEN WE COME UP against a difficult situation or quandary, especially an issue that has become a common occurrence or source of frustration, it is useful to look at the intervention possible at each stage of the problem. In the following model, consider how each stage of intervention can contribute to the resolution of an ethical issue, both in the present and for the future.

Before: Prior to the situation, what, if anything, could have been done to prevent it from arising in the first place?

During: During the situation, what kinds of responses could be appropriate and potentially effective? Consider that in some instances we would want to delay intervention out of respect for the student's privacy.

After: After the situation has occurred, is there an action that needs to be taken? Walk through each possible scenario and list the probable outcomes, and then decide which has the potential to be most effective (including the option not to take any action).

Possible Outcome for the Teacher: Having considered each stage of intervention, now consider the effects your actions might have for yourself now and in the future.

Possible Outcome for the Student: Consider the possible effects that your actions might have on the student now and in the future. Try to see this from both the student's point of view and your own.

SAMPLE ETHICAL INQUIRY: ATTENTION-SEEKING STUDENT

You are leading a Yoga intensive, and one of the participants is consistently hogging the question-and-answer time. Her questions are generally vague and rarely relevant to the material being covered. At times her questions do not seem to be questions at all but opportunities to relate personal stories that are not of interest to the group. You note that the rest of the group becomes restless and begins to shut down as soon as she begins speaking.

Stages of Intervention

Before: At the beginning of the intensive, ask the group whether they would be willing to make these agreements: 1. Internalize questions prior to asking them so that the question is clear and to determine whether the question is relevant to the material being covered. 2. Consider whether the question is of such a personal nature as to not be useful to the rest of the group. If it is, consider approaching the teacher with it after the class is over. 3. Make sure that your question is not the result of not paying attention (repeating a question that has already been answered). Making such agreements with the whole group is a way to provide clear parameters and make your expectations known. It can prevent the need to single out an individual.

During: Assuming you have made asked for agreements at the beginning of the intensive, the student nonetheless continues her behavior. When the student asks a vague question, consider saying, "I don't understand the nature of your question. Would you please spend some time clarifying your question and we will return to you later." When the student asks an irrelevant question, consider saying, "With all due respect, that question does not pertain to the material we are covering right now." If the student begins to digress into long personal monologues, consider saying, "Excuse me, could you please tell me what your question is?" If the student continually has her hand up during question time, simply ignore her by calling on other students.

After: If the behavior continues, you may want to make a general announcement asking people to be sensitive during the question-and-answer time to allow everyone time for their questions. Some people are extroverted and tend to dominate question time. You might ask these people to make it a practice to internalize their questions. Others tend to be wallflowers during question times. You might ask these people (who have generally thought a great deal about their questions) to consider sharing their questions more with the group. When a student continues to display attention-getting behavior in a way that is disrupting the learning process for the rest of the group, as a last resort you might take the student aside and gently suggest that she spend one class (or one day) internalizing her questions (i.e., thinking about but not asking questions out loud). Frequently this kind of behavior has to do with the student's inability to contain her process appropriately. When I have had to use this strategy, I have framed it as wanting to see the student develop a greater trust in her own inner reference system.

Possible Outcome for the Teacher: By limiting questions to those that are relevant, I can focus more clearly on the material I wish to cover. My energy is liberated to meet the needs of the group, rather than being caught up in the needs of one person. By being clear about etiquette for asking questions, I prevent possible frustration and irritation, both for myself and the other students.

Possible Outcome for the Student: The student may learn more about her process of inquiry and learn to seek an internal reference for her questions, thus increasing her independence. She may also be learning how to practice awareness about the needs of others and to be considerate in not hogging the teachers' time.

Sample Ethical Inquiries

Now, by yourself, with a colleague, or as a part of a group discussion, consider how you might approach the following situations. Consider each ethical quandary in terms of the stages of intervention and the potential outcomes of various actions.

Injured by Another Teacher: A student of another teacher comes into your class and reports that he has been badly injured. He relates the details of the incident, and it appears that the teacher was at fault. He no longer wishes to study with this teacher. The teacher is a colleague at a center where you also teach.

Criticizing Other Teachers or Methods: During your beginning-level Yoga class, a man asks "What do you think about _____ Yoga?" He might be asking about a specific method or style of Yoga. You personally have strong reservations about this method of Yoga. Is there a way to voice your concerns ethically? Is there a way to circumvent the question that places the question firmly back in the student's court?

Questionable Alliances: A celebrity begins attending one of your public Yoga classes. The class is large, and it is difficult even at the best of times to give everyone the personal attention you would like. The celebrity student makes it clear that he expects special attention. You also perceive that forming an alliance with this student may be advantageous to your career (for example, if he owns a video company).

Teaching Appropriate Levels: You have a job at a local gym, where you teach a regular Yoga class. The director of the gym makes it clear that she would like you to conduct the class at a faster pace and make the content more physically demanding. Although there are several students in the class who could handle a more difficult class, the core of the class is made up of people who have had little physical conditioning, with many suffering mild but chronic back pain. These core students have also been the most loyal and regular attendees.

Gray Zones: A casual acquaintance is suffering from cancer and has heard that Yoga may be of help to her. You kindly offer to give private lessons in her home, and after several months it becomes clear that she is terminally ill. The sessions appear to be of great benefit. Her husband has also attended the sessions to act as a support for his wife and to help her remember the details of each session. Although the husband is not your student, you find yourself thinking about a relationship with him. When the student dies, you have strong fantasies of beginning a relationship with the husband.

Student Lateness: A student regularly arrives late for class. When she enters the classroom, she disrupts the group, taking a place in the front row. After the class, she makes it a habit to stay afterward to ask you many questions.

Romantic Solicitation by a Student: A student whom you find attractive sends you an e-mail asking if you would like to go out for dinner together. You sense that he is interested in pursuing a personal relationship with you.

Student Pressure: You are working with a small, diverse group of beginning students and feel pressured by many of them to teach material that is beyond their current level of practice. You sense that teaching a "harder" class may put you in greater favor and possibly increase your class numbers.

Yoga Class as Social Support: One of your long-standing students has just incurred a series of losses: her husband passed away this year, she has been laid off her job, and her daughter has just been diagnosed with a serious illness. Her attendance at your weekly Yoga class is one of her main sources of social support. However, you observe that she is becoming increasingly frail and have concerns about her safety in keeping up with the rest of the group. You are also concerned that she would experience asking her to attend a different class as a form of rejection and a severance from key friends who currently attend her class. How might you accommodate her situation?

Student with Anorexia: One of your female students is clearly suffering from advanced anorexia, showing signs of severe emaciation, hair loss, and pale complexion. In consulting with other Yoga teachers whose classes she attends, you discover that she is attending two or three classes a day and bicycling around town in between. In your discussions you conclude that she not only has an eating disorder but has clear signs of exercise obsession as well. Her body is so frail that you now have concerns about adjusting her postures because of suspected osteoporosis. You also have serious reservations about the suitability of her attending any Yoga class until she gets clinical help for her disease. Consider what you might do as an individual teacher and also consider a course of action for all the teachers whose classes she attends.

Teaching Family Members: Your mother has asked if she can attend your Yoga classes. Although she has years of self-practice, she has had little formal instruction. Despite this lack of formal instruction, she has dogmatic views on how to do the postures and also how she wishes to be adjusted. When you adjust her postures, she frequently asks you to give her more pressure than you believe would be safe. She seems to have the remarkable ability to reverse the roles with you, so you feel you are becoming *her* student. You become infuriated with her during class, yet at the same time you sense this is a golden opportunity to become closer to your mother and to break through some longstanding patterns in your relationship. Consider some options for a plan of action.

Inappropriate Dress: An attractive young woman begins taking Yoga classes at your center. You've noticed that her Yoga clothes are so skimpy that her breasts frequently pop out of her yoga tops during inverted postures such as Headstand (Salamba Sirsasana), and her low-rise yoga pants seem designed to prove that she is a genuine redhead! You find yourself avoiding adjusting her postures and observe that a number of young men in the class seem to be distracted by her presence. Consider an intervention plan for before, during, and after the situation with this student and a plan for addressing the general dress code for your class. If you are a center director, also consider the dress code of the teachers.

Late Payments: You've just begun teaching your first beginning-level Yoga class, and most of the attendees are friends. Even though you requested that students preregister and prepay for the course, you are now into the third week of the course and a number of your student-friends have still not paid for their classes. You feel uncomfortable confronting personal friends with your financial concerns, so you delay doing so. Consider why this situation has arisen. Is your avoidance or delay in addressing these financial concerns contributing to the problem? Consider the deeper reasons why you feel uncomfortable about asking for fair remuneration. How could you ensure fair and prompt payment in the future?

Refunds: Your Yoga brochure has a clearly stated payment policy for class cards (for example, ten classes for $150, which must be used within ten weeks of purchase). You notice that you have a consistent problem with people trying to extend their class cards, even though the time limitation is one of the rationales for the discount in price. When you hold to your position and refuse to give a time extension, a student accuses you of "being too commercial" and says, "I thought Yoga was about being spiritual." Another variation of this problem is the student who does not use a class card during the time limit and requests a refund. How might you reduce the incidence of such unpleasant encounters?

Poaching Students: While you are away on holiday, you ask a colleague to cover your classes. Upon your return you discover that he has actively solicited the students to attend his classes, handing out his own Yoga class schedule at the end of every session. You are disgruntled at what appears to be an overt attempt to steal students from your established group. Consider if you would have felt differently had the teacher made no direct solicitation but several students had enjoyed the substitute classes so much that they decided to change teachers. Examine the ethics of each situation.

Mixing Professional and Personal: A longtime Yoga student helps you with the finances to expand your Yoga center. Her investment is substantial, allowing you to buy the building you once leased and to make the renovations that allow you to increase your class schedule. Over the years, the student has become a casual personal friend, but since making her financial investment she has begun to ask you for professional help in the form of private lessons and is offended when you ask for payment. Additionally she becomes very upset when you decline her social invitations or when she indicates that she would like a more personal friendship with you. What might you have done prior to accepting her help to avoid the complications that have now arisen between you? Is there anything you can do now to ameliorate your current conflict?

APPENDIX:

YOGA SUTRA OF PATANJALI TRANSLATIONS SOURCED

Swami Venkatesananda, *Enlightened Living: A New Interpretative Translation of the Yoga Sutra of Maharsi Patanjali*, 3d. ed. (Sebastopol, CA: Anahata Press, 1999).

Alistair Shearer, *The Yoga Sutras of Patanjali* (New York: Bell Tower, 2002).

T. K.V. Desikachar, *Patanjali's Yogasutras* (New Delhi: Affiliated East-West Press Pvt. Ltd., in association with Rupa and Co., 1987).

Barbara Stoler Miller, *Yoga: Discipline of Freedom* (New York: Bantam Books, 1995).

Kofi Busia, *The Gift, The Prayer, The Offering* (Oxford: Oxford Ashram Publications, 1984).

Sutra Cited

Part I
The Sacred Role of Teacher

Sutra 1.1 (translation by Venkatesananda)

Now, when a sincere seeker approaches an enlightened teacher, with the right attitude of discipleship (viz., free of preconceived notions and prejudices, and full of intelligent faith and receptivity) and with the right spirit of inquiry, at the right time and the right place, communication of yoga takes place.

What Is a Yoga Teacher?

Sutra 1.13 (translation by Shearer)
The practice of yoga is the commitment to become established in the state of freedom.

Yoga Teacher as Mentor

Sutra 1.40 (translation by Shearer)
The sovereignty of the mind that is settled extends from the smallest of the small to the greatest of the great.

Ethics and Ethical Behavior

Sutra II.29 (translation by Venkatesananda)
Discipline, observances, posture, exercise of the life-force, introversion of attention, concentration, meditation and illumination (at-one-ment) are the eight limbs of yoga or the direct realization of oneness. Hence, these limbs should all be practiced together, intelligently, so that the impurities of all the physical, vital and psychological limbs may be eliminated.

Archetypes: How the Teacher Lives in the Student's Mind

Sutra 1.4 (translation by Desikachar)
In the absence of the state of mind called Yoga the ability to understand the object is simply replaced by the mind's conception of that object or by a total lack of comprehension.

Yoga Teacher as Healer

Sutra II.15 (translation by Shearer)
Life is uncertain, change causes fear, and latent impressions bring pain— all is indeed suffering to one who has developed discriminations.

Yoga Teacher as Priest

Sutra II.26 (translation by Shearer)
Ignorance is destroyed by the undisturbed discrimination between the Self and the world.

Yoga Teacher as Parent

Sutra II.24 (translation by Shearer)
It is ignorance of our real nature that causes the Self to be obscured.

Yoga Teacher as Lover

Sutra II.38 (translation by Busia)
Through communion with God, one becomes truly strong.

Transference, Countertransference, Projection, Adoration, and Emulation

Sutra I.4 (translation by Venkatesananda)
At other times, when yoga does not happen and when the mind is busily occupied with the movement, there is a cloud of confusion in the undivided, homogeneous intelligence. In the shadow of that cloud, there arises false identification or cognition of the movement of the mind-fragment and hence

distorted understanding. The single concept or idea or the single movement of thought is mistaken as the totality.

Healthy Boundaries

Sutra II.35 (translation by Desikachar)
The more considerate one is, the more one stimulates friendly feelings among all in one's presence.

Sexual Ethics

Sutra II.34 (translation by Shearer)
Negative feelings, such as violence, are damaging to life, whether we act upon them ourselves or cause or condone them in others. They are born of greed, anger or delusion, and may be slight, moderate or intense. Their fruit is endless ignorance and suffering. To remember this is to cultivate the opposite.

The Teacher's Social, Personal, and Sexual Needs

Sutra II. 37 (translation by Shearer)
When we are firmly established in integrity, all riches present themselves freely.

PART II:

The Ethics of Professional Yoga Practice

Sutra 1.33 (translation by Shearer)
The mind becomes clear and serene when the qualities of the heart are culti-vated: friendliness towards the joyful, compassion towards their suffering, happiness towards the pure, and impartiality towards the impure.

Teacher Training

Sutra 1.14 (translation by Desikachar)
It is only when the correct practice is followed for a long time, without inter-ruptions and with a quality of positive attitude and eagerness, that it can suc-ceed. (The goal of practice is to bring about a change in the quality of the mind. When practice is pursued for a long time without interruption, and when the results, good or bad, do not bring about elation or dejection, then the practice is considered to be deeply rooted and bound to succeed).

Training Programs

Sutra 1.13 (translation by Shearer)
The practice of yoga is the commitment to become established in the state of freedom.

Certification

Sutra 1.21 (translation by Desikachar)
The more intense the faith and the effort, the closer the goal.

The Dangers of Charisma and the Pitfalls of Fame

Sutra 1.8 (translation by Desikachar)
Misapprehension is that comprehension which is taken to be correct until more favorable conditions reveal the actual nature of the object.

Medical Concerns and Making Unfair Claims

Sutra III.46 (translation by Venkatesananda)
What constitutes perfection of the body? Beauty, grace, strength, and adamantine firmness.

Class Numbers

Sutra II.37 (translation by Shearer)
When we are firmly established in integrity, all riches present themselves freely.

Ethical Class Structures

Sutra II.36 (translation by Shearer)
When we are firmly established in truthfulness, action accomplishes its desired end.

Class Levels

Sutra II.46 (translation by Venkatesananda)
The posture of the body during the practice of contemplation and at other times, as also the posture of the mind (or attitude to life) should be firm and pleasant.

How We Communicate with Students

Sutra II.36 (translation by Desikachar)
One who shows a high degree of right communication, will not fail in his actions.

Adjustments and Touching

Sutra II.47 (translation by Shearer)
[Asanas] are mastered when all effort is relaxed and the mind is absorbed in the infinite.

The Power of Words

Sutra II.36 (translation by Venkatesananda)
When there is firm grounding in the perception of what is, or of truth, it is seen that an action and reaction, seed and its fruits, or cause and result are related to each other; and the clear vision of intelligence becomes directly aware of this relationship. (Or, one's words are fruitful.)

Codes of Etiquette

Sutra II.30 (translation by Desikachar)
Yama comprises:
1. Consideration towards all living things, especially those who are innocent, in difficulty, or worse off than we are.
2. Right communications through speech, writings, gesture and action.
3. Non-covetousness or the ability to resist a desire for that which does not belong to us.

4. Moderation in all our actions.
5. Non-greediness or the ability to accept only what is appropriate.

Boundaries

Sutra IV.15 (translation by Shearer)
Two similar objects appear differently, depending upon the different mental states of the observer.

The Ethics of Money

Sutra II.37 (translation by Busia)
Through the devoted practice of not taking things, the greatest treasures are made manifest.

Appropriate Dress for the Teacher

Sutra II.40 (translation by Desikachar)
When cleanliness is developed it reveals what needs to be constantly maintained and what is eternally clean. What decays is external. What does not is deep within us.

Confidentiality

Sutra II.36 (translation by Stoler Miller)
When one abides in truthfulness, activity and its fruition are grounded in the truth.

Speaking About Other Teachers or Methods

Sutra 1.8 (translation by Busia)
Incorrect knowledge is a false understanding not based on the true nature of what is perceived.

Ethical Codes

Sutra II.31 (translation by Stoler Miller)
These universal moral principles [yamas], unrestricted by conditions of birth, place, time or circumstance, are the great vow of yoga.

NOTES

PART I

1. Barbara Stoler Miller, trans., *Yoga: Discipline of Freedom* (New York: Bantam Books, 1995), 53.

2. Kylea Taylor, *The Ethics of Caring: Honoring the Web of Life in Our Professional Healing Relationships* (Santa Cruz, CA: Hanford Mead Publishers, 1995), 10.

3. Often referred to as the Golden Rule, Jesus' Sermon on the Mount has its corollary in the Talmud, the Koran, and the Analects of Confucius.

4. Rachel Naomi Remen, quoted in Taylor, *Ethics of Caring*, 3.

5. *The Random House Dictionary of the English Language*, unabridged 2nd ed., s.v. "master."

6. Donna Farhi, *Bringing Yoga to Life: The Everyday Practice of Enlightened Living* (San Francisco: HarperSanFrancisco, 2003), 175–87.

7. Yoga Nidra is an ancient Tantric practice that involves profoundly deep states of relaxation in which one inquires into the nature of one's true identity.

8. Phillip Moffitt, "Good Fences Make for Good Relations," *Yoga Journal*, May/June 2005, 120.

9. Ibid.

10. Peter Rutter, *Sex in the Forbidden Zone: When Men in Power—Therapists, Doctors, Clergy, Teachers and Others—Betray Women's Trust* (Los Angeles: Jeremy Tarcher, 1989), 21.

11. Ibid., 41.

Part II

1. An excellent resource for Yoga teachers who want to learn about the ethics of teaching is *The Elements of Teaching* by James M. Banner, Jr., and Harold C. Cannon (New Haven: Yale University Press, 1997).

2. The word *mudra* has a number of meanings. In this context, it connotes a "seal" or body "lock" for containing and directing pranic energy.

3. Yoga therapy is a contemporary term to describe what yoga adepts have done for centuries: adapting and tailoring a yoga practice to ameliorate or cure a specific health condition, injury, or disease. Although some practitioners of Yoga therapy are medical doctors or physical therapists, many do not have a medical license but have had specialized training for working with a particular population of students. The use of Yoga as a therapy includes, but is not limited to, the treatment of asthma, back pain, cardiovascular disease, depression, diabetes, eating disorders, high blood pressure, muscular dystrophy, obesity, and repetitive strain injuries.

   The International Association of Yoga Therapists (IAYT) defines *Yoga therapy* as providing "instruction in yogic practices and teachings to prevent or alleviate pain and suffering and their root causes. It is best taught one-on-one to address the unique matrix of conditions and aspirations of the student. Practices may include, but are not limited to, asana, pranayama, meditation, sound and chanting, personal ritual, and prayer. Teaching may also include, but is not limited to, directed study, discussion, and lifestyle counseling. Yoga therapy may address any of the dimensions of life. In the classical tradition, these are the *panca kosha*, or five sheaths, of the human being. In contemporary terms, these may be approximated as the anatomical, physiological, emotional, intellectual, and spiritual dimensions." For more information about IAYT, visit www.iayt.org.

4. Ethical Guidelines for Yoga Teachers from the Yoga Research and Education Center (YREC), copyright © 2000 by the Yoga Research and Education Center. YREC gladly grants permission to reproduce these guidelines upon written request and providing that their copyright notice is reproduced along with the guidelines. Visit www.yrec.org for more information.

APPRECIATIONS

GRATEFUL ACKNOWLEDGEMENT is made to the following for permission to reprint previously published material:

Affiliated East-West Press Private, Ltd.: Excerpts from *Patanjali's Yogasutras: An Introduction*, by T. K. V. Desikachar; copyright © 1987 by T. K. V. Desikachar; reprinted by permission.

Anahata Press: Excerpts from *Enlightened Living: A New Interpretative Translation of the Yoga Sutra of Maharsi Patanjali*, by Swami Venkatesananda; copyright © 1999 by Chiltern Yoga Trust; reprinted by permission; www.nondual.com.

Bell Tower, a division of Random House, Inc.: Excerpts from *The Yoga Sutras of Patanjali*, by Alistair Shearer; copyright © 1982 by Alistair Shearer; reprinted by permission.

Oxford Ashram Publications: Excerpts from *The Gift, The Prayer, The Offering: A Translation of the Yoga Sutras of Patanjali*, by Kofi Busia; copyright © 1984 by Kofi Busia; reprinted with permission; www.kofibusia.org.

ABOUT THE AUTHOR

DONNA FARHI has practiced Yoga for thirty years and has taught internationally for over two decades. She travels the world teaching Yoga and training others to teach. Donna has been the asana columnist for *Yoga International* and *Yoga Journal,* and is the author of *The Breathing Book*; *Yoga Mind, Body and Spirit*; and *Bringing Yoga to Life*. Born in the United States, she now resides in New Zealand.

For information about Donna's Yoga classes, workshops, and teacher trainings, visit www.donnafarhi.co.nz.

FROM THE PUBLISHER

RODMELL PRESS publishes books on yoga, Buddhism, aikido, and Taoism. In the Bhagavadgita it is written, "Yoga is skill in action." It is our hope that our books will help individuals develop a more skillful practice—one that brings peace to their daily lives and to the earth.

We thank those whose support, encouragement, and practical advise sustain us in our efforts. In particular, we are grateful to Reb Anderson, B. K. S. Iyengar, Wendy Palmer, and Yvonne Rand for their inspiration.

To request a catalog or receive e-announcements about new titles, contact us at:

(510) 841-3123 or (800) 841-3123
(510) 841-3123 (fax)
info@rodmellpress.com
www.rodmellpress.com

Rodmell Press is distributed to the trade by Publishers Group West:

(800) 788-3123
(510) 528-5511 (sales fax)
info@pgw.com

INDEX

adjustments and touching. *See also* sexual
impropriety by teachers
  adjusting clothing, 126–127
  asking permission, 37–38, 90
  injury from, 91
  pitfalls to fame and, 65
  sexualizing, avoiding, 45
  stopping when asked, 90–91
  value of, 89–90
adoration, 24–25, 35, 64–65
amplification for large groups, 79–80
anorexia, 150–151
apologies, 94
archetypes of the teacher. *See also* roles of
the teacher
  healer, 22–24
  impact of, 20–22
  lover, 30–31
  parent figure, 26–28
  priest, 25–26
Ashtanga Yoga, 9, 11, 137
atman, 16
authority vs. authoritarianism, 89

body odor, 127
boundaries, 37–47, 105–109
  before and after class, 106–107, 108–109,
    112
  on attention seeking, 107–108, 146–148,
    149
  "being spiritual" and, 107
  for class structures, 83
  codes of etiquette, 94–104
  as container for the process, 37, 83

educating students about, 37–38
  enmeshment, 42–43
  friendship and, 40, 41–42
  modeled by teacher, 105
  necessary distance, 39–41
  pedagogical models and, 38–39
  private space for teachers, 44
  for questions, 97–98, 105–106, 146–148
  questions to ask about, 43
  sexual ethics and, 44–47
  starting and finishing on time, 107
  students pushing, 29–30
  transgressions of etiquette, 99–101
boycotting, 5, 135–136
Bringing Yoga to Life, 34

caring for vs. taking care of, 26–28
CD, about, 178
certification. *See* training and certification
charisma. *See* fame and charisma
class numbers, 75–80
  amplification for large groups, 79–80
  demand for senior teachers and, 77–78
  experience levels and, 75–76
  money issues and, 76, 78–79, 86–87
  safety and, 75–76, 77
  for special-needs students, 87
  for workshops and intensives, 76–79
class structures and levels, 80–88
  class numbers and, 75–76
  container created by boundaries, 83
  drop-in students, 80–81, 82
  exceeding teacher's practice, 85–86
  mixing student levels, avoiding, 80–81

90 percent-10 percent rule, 85
partial attendance, 82, 83
prerequisites, advantages of, 81–82
teaching at the students' level, 84–85, 86,
    88, 149, 150
for workshops and intensives, 82
cleanliness, 127
codes of ethics, 134–139
    boycotting and, 5, 135–136
    efforts to establish, 134–136
    formal, lacking for profession, 134
    handling complaints and, 140, 142–143
    in the Yoga Sutra, 134, 137
    from YREC, 137–139, 166
codes of etiquette, 94–104
    asking questions, 97–98, 146–148
    communicating creatively, 103
    handling transgressions, 99–101
    honoring inner perceptions, 96–97
    leaving class, 98–99
    necessity of, 94–95
    promptness, 27–28, 96, 100, 149
    silent focus, 98
    Yoga Tree studio example, 103–104
communication with students. See also
        adjustments and touching
    about other teachers or methods,
        131–132, 148
    apologies, 94
    authority vs. authoritarianism, 89
    confidentiality, 25, 128–131, 132–133
    constructive critique, 92–93
    feedback, welcoming, 91
    foul language, 127–128
    popularity vs. true worth, 63
    saying you don't know, 73–74
    word choices and meanings, 93–94
community (sangha)
    reverence and respect instilled by, 3
    unethical behavior overlooked by, 4–5, 65
compassion (ahimsa), 11, 12
complaints, handling, 91, 112–113, 140–143
confidentiality, 25, 128–131, 132–133
constraints (yamas and niyamas), 9, 11–13,
    137
contentment (santosha), 11, 13
countertransference, 34

disciplined energy (tapas), 11, 13
disenchantment with the teacher, 35–36
dress, appropriate
    for students, 126–127, 151
    for teachers, 123–126

eight limbs of Yoga, 9, 11, 17, 55, 137, 156
emulation of the teacher, 35
enmeshment, 42–43
ethical inquiries
    about, 6
    appropriate intervention, 73
    attention-seeking students, 107–108,
        146–148, 149
    boundaries before and after class, 108–109
    business viability and integrity, 118–119
    changing monetary agreements, 116–117
    complexity of, 143
    confidentiality, 132–133
    dress, inappropriate, 125–126, 151
    having a supervisor, 49
    late payments, 115–116, 151–152
    mixing professional and personal,
        152–153
    pedestal, putting teacher on, 24–25
    private space from students, 44
    pushing boundaries, 29–30
    referral for medical help, 69–70
    refund policies, 118–119, 152
    sample inquiries, 148–152
    saying you don't know, 73–74
    setting safe parameters, 102
    sexual conquest, 31–33
    speaking about students, 133
    special-needs students, 87, 150
    student safety, 68–69
    substitute teachers, 88
    training program scam, 58–60
    visiting teachers, 142–143
ethical issues in teaching. See also ethics of
        teacher–student relationships
    adjustments and touching, 89–91, 126–127
    boundaries, 105–109, 112
    charisma and fame, 63–66, 77–78
    class numbers, 75–80, 86–87
    class structures and levels, 75–76, 80–88,
        149, 150

codes of ethics, 134–139, 140, 142–143
codes of etiquette, 94–104
communication with students, 63, 73–74,
    88–94, 127–133
confidentiality, 25, 128–131, 132–133
dress, 123–127, 151
educational resources for, 52
handling complaints, 91, 112–113, 140–143
medical, health, and safety, 66–76, 77, 102
money, 76, 78–79, 86–87, 110–123,
    135–136
poaching students, 152
scope of, 51–52, 53, 143
speaking of other teachers or methods,
    131–133, 148
training and certification, 5, 54–62
workbook for resolving, 145–153
The Ethics of Caring, 17
ethics of teacher-student relationships. *See
    also* ethical issues in teaching
    definitions of ethics, 17–18
    external locus for, 18–19
    internal locus for, 18
    questions to ask, 19–20
    Yoga Sutra and, 17
external locus for ethics, 18–19

fame and charisma
    adoration and, 24–25, 35, 64–65
    class numbers and, 77–78
    pitfalls to fame, 64–66
    popularity vs. true worth, 63–64
    questionable alliances, 149
Farhi, Donna
    about, 169
    boycotts by, 5, 135
    early training in Yoga, 1–3
    reasons for writing this book, 3, 5
    sacred role of teachers for, 7–8
    work in ethics, 4–5
finances. *See* money issues
financial assistance, 120–123
finishing class on time, 107
friendship, teacher-student, 40, 41–42
Frost, Taffy, 103

"Good Fences Make for Good Relations," 42

healer, teacher as, 22–24
heart, qualities of (brahmavihara), 16, 159
Hittleman, Richard, 1

injuries. *See* medical, health, and safety
    issues
inquiries. *See* ethical inquiries
internal locus for ethics, 18

Jesus, 17–18, 165

laws and legal issues, 52, 65, 130, 141,
    142, 144
levels. *See* class structures and levels
lover, teacher as, 30–31

medical, health, and safety issues
    adjustments and touching, 91
    anorexia, 150–151
    appropriate intervention, 73
    class numbers and safety, 75–76, 77
    diagnosis, 66
    injury by another teacher, 148
    items to consider, 67–68
    mental and emotional, 67–69, 71, 72
    referrals, 69–70, 71–72
    setting safe parameters, 102
    unfounded claims, 66, 70–71
mentor, teacher as, 15–17
Miller, Richard, 57
Moffit, Phillip, 42
money issues, 110–123
    asking too little, 111–112
    boycotting, 135–136
    business viability and integrity, 118–119
    changing agreements, 116–117
    class numbers and, 76, 78–79, 86–87
    complaints about payment, 112–113
    donations, 110
    financial assistance, 120–123
    late payments, 115–116, 151–152
    mixing professional and personal,
        152–153
    prepayment and preregistration, 114–115
    refund policies, 115, 118–119, 152
    spiritual conceptions and, 110–111
    teaching without compensation, 123

mudra, 65, 166

niyamas and yamas, 9, 11–13, 137
not grasping (aparigraha), 11, 12
not stealing (asteya), 11, 12, 106, 112

observancs (yamas and niyamas), 9, 11–13,
    137
On Defining Spirit, 18

parent figure, teacher as, 26–28
Patanjali. *See* Yoga Sutra of Patanjali
pedestal, putting teacher on, 24–25, 35
poaching students, 152
priest, teacher as, 25–26
projection, 28, 34–35
promptness, 27–28, 96, 100, 149
Publishers Group West, 171
purity (shaucha), 11, 13

qualities of heart (brahmavihara), 16, 159
question-and-answer issues, 97–98,
    105–106, 146–148

refund policies, 115, 118–119, 152
Remen, Rachel Naomi, 18
restraints (yamas and niyamas), 9, 11–13,
    137
Richard Hittleman's Yoga, 1
Rodmell Press, 171
roles of the teacher. *See also* archetypes of
    the teacher
    mentor, 15–17
    professional vs. private behavior, 10
    sacred, 7–9
    Yoga as a way of living and, 9–15
    Yoga master, 22
Rutter, Peter, 44–45

sacred role of teacher, 7–9
scholarships, 121–122
self-disclosure in teaching, 24–25
self-study (swadhyaya), 11, 13
Sex in the Forbidden Zone, 44–45
sexual impropriety by students
    conquest, 31–33
    in dress, 126, 151

seeking self-worth, 30–31
transference, 33–34
sexual impropriety by teachers. *See also*
    adjustments and touching
abuse defined, 45
countertransference, 34
as disempowering, 33
in dress, 123–126
gray areas, 46–47, 149
handling complaints, 140–143
legal issues, 65, 141, 142, 144
"master" title and, 22
overlooked by Yoga community, 4–5, 65
pitfalls to fame and, 65
power and, 44–45, 47
sexual ethics and, 44–46
teacher's needs and, 47–49
sexual propriety (brahmacharya), 11, 12
silence, etiquette of, 98
size of classes. *See* class numbers
special-needs students
    anorexic student, 150–151
    class as social support for, 150
    class numbers for, 87
    information needed from, 67
    questions raised by work with, 23
    screening process for, 67–68
structures. *See* class structures and levels
substitute teachers, 88
surrender to God (ishvarapranidhana),
    11, 13

Taylor, Kylea, 17, 18
teacher–student relationship
    adoration and emulation, 24–25, 35,
        64–65
    archetypes in student's mind, 20–31
    boundaries, 29–30, 37–47
    countertransference, 34
    disenchantment, 35–36
    enmeshment, 42–43
    friendship, 40, 41–42
    healthy, determining, 49–50
    mentor role of the teacher, 15–17
    professional vs. private behavior, 10
    projection, 28, 34–35
    sacred role of teacher, 7–9

sexual conquest by student, 31–33
teacher's needs and, 47–49
transference, 33–34
Yoga as a way of living and, 9–15
touching. *See* adjustments and touching;
    sexual impropriety by students; sexual
    impropriety by teachers
training and certification, 54–62
    certification issues, 54, 60–62
    character of teachers and, 60–61
    choosing a program, 54–58, 61, 62
    prerequisites for programs, 56–57
    quality of training faculty and, 56
    reflected value of the community, 57
    researching programs, 57–58
    scope of training, 54–55
    standards lacking for, 5, 54
    time required for, 55–56
    training program scam, 58–60
    trainings from Donna Farhi, 169
transference, 33–34
truthfulness (satya), 11, 12

unfounded claims, 66, 70–71

workbook for resolving ethical issues
    attention-seeking example, 146–148
    sample ethical inquiries, 148–153
    working model, 145–146
work-study arrangements, 121, 122

yamas and niyamas, 9, 11–13, 137
Yoga Nidra, 40, 78, 165
Yoga Research and Education Center
    (YREC), 137–139, 166

Yoga Sutra of Patanjali
    described, 11
    ethics and, 17, 52, 137
    yamas and niyamas in, 11–13, 137
    I.1 (teacher–student relationship), 7,
        155–156
    I.4 (state of mind called Yoga), 20, 33, 156,
        157–158
    I.8 (misapprehension), 63, 131, 160, 163
    I.13 (commitment to freedom), 9, 54, 156,
        159
    I.14 (long-time practice), 54, 159
    I.21 (faith and effort), 60, 159
    I.33 (qualities of heart), 16, 159
    I.40 (sovereignty of mind), 15, 156
    II.15 (all is suffering), 22, 157
    II.24 (ignorance obscures Self), 26, 157
    II.26 (ignorance destroyed by discrimina-
        tion), 25, 157
    II.29 (eight limbs of Yoga), 17, 156
    II.30 (yamas), 94, 161–162
    II.31 (yamas), 10, 134, 163
    II.34 (negative feelings), 44, 158
    II.35 (considerateness), 37, 158
    II.36 (right communication), 80, 88, 92,
        128, 160, 161, 162
    II.37 (non-covetousness), 47, 74, 110, 158,
        160, 162
    II.38 (moderation), 30, 157
    II.40 (cleanliness), 123, 162
    II.46 (posture), 160
    II.47 (mastery of asanas), 89, 161
    III.46 (perfection of the body), 66, 84, 160
    IV.15 (appearances and mental states), 105,
        162
Yoga therapy, 66, 166
Yoga Tree studio etiquette, 103–104

ABOUT THE CD:

HOLDING A HEART IN OUR HANDS

DONNA FARHI EXPLORES the meaning of the teacher–student relationship and importance of ethics in "Holding a Heart in Our Hands," her keynote address to yoga teachers and students at Yoga Spirit 2002, a conference held in Lake George, New York. It is intended for personal listening, to be shared with colleagues, and to be used in Yoga teacher-training courses to inspire questions, thoughtful inquiry, and lively discussion. 74:20 minutes.